for all those seeking hope

Praise for Kate Fagan's

WHAT MADE MADDY RUN

"Gripping and universal."　　—Trevor Noah, *The Daily Show*

"A poignant study of the converging pressures of mental illness, college athletics, and social media."
　　　　　　　　　　　　　　—Carlos Lozada, *Washington Post*

"*What Made Maddy Run* dives deep...Fagan's ability to take us inside those intimate and painful moments makes this narrative compelling...For Maddy's words alone, read this book. It is a comprehensive, essential, and well-written piece about mental health, as well as a small step toward reducing the stigma around anxiety and depression."
　　　　　　　　　　　—Erin McCarthy, *Philadelphia Inquirer*

"With immense empathy, Fagan shares insights particular to student athletes, but presents them in universally accessible language and connects with the nonathlete through vivid examples...Fagan removes the filters her subject so carefully applied and demonstrates with sensitivity and compassion the urgent need to understand and address a deadly problem."
　　　　　　　　　　　　　　　—Jen Forbus, *Shelf Awareness*

"A provocative and thoughtful look at a student-athlete suicide that rocked the nation—but didn't, until now, actually help inform the nation. A labor of love and prevention by Kate Fagan, and Maddy's family and friends."

—Stephen Fried, author of *Thing of Beauty*

"It is impossible not to be affected by Holleran's heart-wrenching story. An appropriate (if difficult) read for current and future college athletes, their coaches, and their parents."

—Sara Holder, *Library Journal*

"Throughout telling Maddy's story, Fagan does an exceptional job weaving in her experience of venturing into Maddy's troubled past...She delivers the sequence of events in such a heartfelt but very real way."

—Caitlyn Pilkington, *Women's Running*

"A compassionate and frank look at depression and the social pressure faced by many college students as seen through the eyes of one young woman." —*Kirkus Reviews*

"Holleran seems so alive on the page; her messages and Fagan's prose create someone who seems a real, living thing, so much so that by the end, this reader was rooting for her to talk to someone." —Johanna Gretschel, *FloTrack*

WHAT MADE MADDY RUN

The Secret Struggles and
Tragic Death of an All-American Teen

KATE FAGAN

BACK BAY BOOKS

Little, Brown and Company

New York   Boston   London

Back Bay Books / Little, Brown and Company
Hachette Book Group
1290 Avenue of the Americas, New York, NY 10104
littlebrown.com

Originally published in hardcover by Little, Brown and Company, August 2017
First Back Bay paperback edition, July 2018

Back Bay Books is an imprint of Little, Brown and Company, a division of Hachette Book Group, Inc. The Back Bay Books name and logo are trademarks of Hachette Book Group, Inc.

The publisher is not responsible for websites (or their content) that are not owned by the publisher.

The Hachette Speakers Bureau provides a wide range of authors for speaking events. To find out more, go to hachettespeakersbureau.com or call (866) 376-6591.

Portions of this book are based on "Split/Image" by Kate Fagan, originally published on espnW.com on May 7, 2015. Copyright © 2015 by ESPN, Inc.

Emoji icons provided by EmojiOne (emojione.com)

ISBN 978-0-316-35654-1 (hc) / 978-0-316-35652-7 (pb)
LCCN 2017942319

10 9 8

LSC-C

Printed in the United States of America

Contents

Foreword

By Alison Overholt, Editor in Chief, *ESPN The Magazine* and espnW

I remember the first time Kate and I talked about what it would mean to tell Madison Holleran's story. It was a cold January day, and we sat across from each other at a small table in a crowded mall, so deep in conversation that we barely noticed when the dull roar of lunchtime white noise faded to emptiness as everyone else returned to work. We just kept talking.

It was a *big* conversation—you know, one where you feel the goose bumps start to rise on your skin because you know you're getting close to something important. Kate had written breakthrough stories for espnW and *ESPN The Magazine,* particularly about the glass ceiling women coaches face in the world of elite college sports, but she was determined to make an even bigger impact. I was contemplating returning to ESPN to become editor in chief of espnW, and, like Kate, I was hungry. Her current and my future boss, espnW founder Laura Gentile, had suggested we spend some time together talking about the possibilities.

There was something happening in the world—an awakening of sorts—and we were eagerly dissecting it over now-cold cups of nondescript coffee. But it was more than that—more than simple awareness, or interest. A sense of urgency, perhaps. A feeling that change surrounding the way we talk about and think about and encounter women in the world was brewing. After decades of (often maddeningly) slow and steady progress in the form of policy changes and polite conversations about diversity and equality across business, politics, and, yes, even sports, it felt like the right time.

Even as we discussed witnessing these changes in the world, Kate and I spoke of our sense that in sports journalism, we weren't yet seeing the larger reality reflected in the pages of the pieces we produced or the hours of video journalism we consumed. Where were the girls and women in the bylines of the stories, and as central characters in the narratives they told?

Great narrative journalism has long been about helping us to understand universal truths of the world by grounding big ideas in the stories of real people. I believe that the way we tell these stories can very literally change the way we experience the world. If only boys and men are central characters within complicated subjects, then male stories are universal, while girls' and women's stories remain singular, peculiar. Women's stories the exception; men's stories the rule.

So this is what Kate and I talked about that day over coffee. The overwhelming need we each felt to change the narrative.

And though it is certainly true that everyone has a story, it is also true that some stories help us learn more, grow more. Some stories simply touch us more deeply as they reach right into our hearts, settle there, and never leave.

So that day we talked, by way of example, about a tiny newspaper article. The briefest of summaries of what must have been the deepest of tragedies. Madison Holleran, a young track athlete at the University of Pennsylvania, had died by suicide. Her friends and peers were stunned, several commenting in their confusion that her life was "perfect." Not *seemed* but *was* perfect, as evidenced by the beautifully curated Instagram feed to which she frequently posted, documenting each wonderful moment after the next. Kate and I talked about her. What had she been going through, unseen and unheard, behind all those filters? How much do each of us sift out our struggles and pare away personal truths each day as we work to present a more perfect vision for critique by a social media–fueled world?

We kept talking.

Madison's story was of a life not yet fully lived, a young female athlete facing struggles that, while unique and specific to her particular experiences, could take readers on a universal journey. This, we said, was the kind of story that espnW should bring into the world—big, beautiful, complex, painful, powerful stories, with women and girls as central figures, told through the prism of sports, by writers who care enough to tell them the right way. Writers like Kate.

Sixteen months later, after Maddy's family opened their lives and their hearts to Kate, her story was published by espnW and then in *ESPN The Magazine,* with a companion video feature that ran on ESPN.com and on *SportsCenter.* It was and remains the most read feature in espnW's history, and the most watched video feature in the history of ESPN .com. That story, "Split Image," changed the conversation. At our company, certainly, but in many ways in sports media more broadly and now, with the publication of this book, we hope in the world at large, too. When we read Maddy's story, we feel that we know her. Many of us *are* Maddy, but for the grace of a few decisions or moments of support that placed us on a different path, to a different outcome.

And now here is her fuller story, along with the personal essays and explorations around mental illness that Kate has so thoughtfully crafted in the months since that original publication. It is a powerful and moving work, and one that espnW is honored to have played a role in developing and supporting. It will start conversations—important conversations— about athletes, yes, but more than that, about young people who struggle. With pressure. With illness. With life.

The book you hold in your hands is a special work, by a special writer. Read it. Think about it. Talk about it. Share it. Be a part of changing the narrative.

WHAT MADE
MADDY
RUN

Author's Note

I first met the Holleran family in the summer of 2014, six months after Madison's death. We sat at their kitchen table and I told them I hoped to be able to earn their trust and promised to do justice to Maddy's story. I hope I have fulfilled that promise. Even while dealing with the greatest pain imaginable, the Holleran family opened their home, and their hearts, to me so that we could tell this story: first as a piece for espnW and *ESPN The Magazine,* and now in this book. They answered my calls and e-mails, passed along the cell phone number of every one of Maddy's friends, and even granted me access to Maddy's computer, including her documents, e-mails, and iMessages. A higher purpose drove their transparency: they didn't want Maddy's death to be an isolated tragedy, but rather a catalyst for change. The Madison Holleran Foundation is already doing work to assist those in crisis, placing a special emphasis on preparing high school seniors for the transition to college, which can often be more challenging than expected. In 2016, New Jersey signed into law the Madison Holleran Prevention Act, requiring that New Jersey colleges provide students with around-the-clock access to mental health services.

The content of every document, e-mail, and text reproduced in this book is real, though I have occasionally changed or abbreviated the name of the sender when I thought it appropriate. Madison's death has already created much heartache, and I took extra precautions so as not to create more.

No premeditated reason exists for why I alternately refer to Madison by both her full name and as Maddy, though it is true to say I felt that, by writing this book, I came to know her—at least in some small way.

CHAPTER 1

Shattered

The night before returning to the University of Pennsylvania for the start of second semester, Madison Holleran broke her iPhone. She was with her whole family at the local TGI Friday's, one of their go-to spots. The iPhone 4 slipped from her hand while she was walking to the car after dinner. She picked it up from the ground and looked at the glass: shattered.

"I can't go back to school with my phone like this," Madison told her dad, Jim.

He smiled. He knew that she couldn't; she depended on her phone. Over the years, father and daughter had spent countless hours in the car together, driving to and from school and practices, Maddy always doing something on her phone, posting photos or sending texts. Jim wasn't big on social media, so he didn't much concern himself with precisely what was capturing Madison's attention. And anyway, she was no different with her phone than any of her friends or anyone else her age—the device was an extension of her hand.

"We'll stop at Verizon on the way back to Penn tomorrow morning," Jim assured his daughter.

The phone did need fixing, but it wasn't *broken*-broken; the problem was cosmetic. So that night, Madison texted with some of her friends, letting them know about the shattered screen—*so annoying, right?*—and making plans for the following afternoon, when she would meet her good friend Ingrid Hung at the Penn women's basketball game. The Quakers were playing Princeton, and one of Maddy's best friends from high school, Jackie Reyneke, was a freshman for the Tigers. Attending the Friday night game meant that Madison had to arrive back on campus three days early. Not ideal. She would have preferred staying at home, spending the weekend with her family in Allendale, New Jersey, working out and sleeping, but she couldn't miss seeing Jackie, with whom she had won two state soccer titles at Northern Highlands, the large public high school they had both attended.

The light tone of Madison's texts camouflaged a truth only a handful of people knew: she dreaded returning to Penn for spring semester. But she was going back. She was continuing to put one foot in front of the other, trying to believe that maybe with the next step she would finally feel solid ground, some semblance of the equilibrium she had known before. At the same time, she couldn't shake the feeling that something had shifted dramatically—something she couldn't quite name. And whatever it was had fundamentally changed how she processed the world.

What was happening to Madison was the inverse of what had happened to her iPhone. She was breaking on the inside.

The next morning, Madison and her dad packed his white Ford Edge. Most of her stuff was still in her dorm room, so all she had was a suitcase and a standing lamp that she had bought while home for Christmas. Her room didn't get much natural light, and she hated the unforgiving overhead glare.

The first stop was at the Verizon on Route 17 in New Jersey. The salesperson took one look at the screen and sent Jim and Maddy to the Apple Store, since that company could likely fix the glass much more cheaply. The stop at Apple in the Garden State Mall was quick. And $200 later, father and daughter were back in the car, heading south to Philadelphia.

The drive was two hours, mostly on Interstate 95, the main corridor between New York City and Philadelphia, a boring stretch of highway broken up only by the occasional exit sign. Jim's mind whirred with everything said and unsaid between them. Just two days earlier, he had attended Maddy's most recent counseling session in the town neighboring Allendale. Before they'd driven over, he'd asked his daughter if she needed to go alone, but she'd said she wanted him there. The session had terrified him. During it, Madison had admitted to suicidal thoughts. He glanced now at his daughter. She was downloading something onto her phone, her brown hair pulled into a ponytail, her eyes focused on the screen.

How have we gotten here? he wondered. Just months ago, she was winning the 800 meters at the New Jersey State Championships, anticipation in the air, the stands filled with a rainbow of school colors, Maddy powering through the finish line as if she could have done yet another lap. In high school, when a practice was too easy, she would come home and run circles around their backyard, actually creating a visible path in the grass.

Now she looked fragile. He couldn't believe he was using that word for her.

Like most parents, Jim prided himself on having solutions when his kids faced problems. Sometimes they took his advice, sometimes they didn't—but at least he had guidance to offer them. Right now, though, Jim had no idea what to say or do. He kept rummaging through his mental toolbox, grabbing at whatever he could. And he kept landing on the same thought: Madison must be going through what Ashley went through. Two years prior, his older daughter had enrolled at Penn State University. She hadn't liked it. She was home almost every weekend, and the family knew she needed to transfer. By sophomore year, she was at the University of Alabama and everything was back to normal.

Maybe that's all Madison needed: a change of scenery. Jim looked again at his daughter. She was so thin, so pale. Energy seemed to be leaking from her as if there was a pinprick nobody could find. Every few minutes, she looked out the window. Jim doubted she was taking in the scene; she seemed to be looking past it. Then she would look back at her phone, continue reconfiguring it.

Second semester will get better, had to get better, Madison thought. If nothing else, through sheer force of will, perhaps she could make it better. And if she told enough people that things were going to go well this time around, said it out loud repeatedly, maybe she could even convince herself.

But one thing had to happen first: She needed to quit track. *Quitting.* Madison had trouble wrapping her mind around that word. She had never quit anything. She was an athlete, had always identified as an athlete. By third grade, she was going to soccer practice multiple times a week — the drills conducted by adults, everything regulated and clearly the start of Madison's march toward continual improvement, both in academics and athletics. Some sort of end goal existed, even if in those earliest years she couldn't quite name it. And then, just before starting middle school, she and her best friend at the time, MJ, had confided in each other that they each wanted to play sports in college. It was her lifelong dream. Yet here she was, just one semester into running track at Penn, wishing she could stop, hoping someone would recognize that she desperately needed to stop.

About halfway down I-95, Madison turned to her dad. "You know I don't want to go back," she said.

"I know," Jim said. "I understand that."

He tightened his grip on the wheel. The road flew beneath the tires. Penn was drawing closer with each passing minute.

"Let's just keep driving," he said. "We could go to North Carolina, to Chapel Hill. We could just keep driving past the exit and you could visit it, see if you like it."

Jim loved Chapel Hill. His sister, Mary, and her husband, Scott, had attended North Carolina. Jim had also gone to school in North Carolina, at High Point University, where he played tennis. The school didn't have the same name recognition, the same clout, as the prestigious East Coast institutions, the vaunted Ivy League, but he had loved his time there. The best four years of his life. He still kept in touch with his college friends.

Madison shook her head. "We can't," she said. "We're having lunch with Ingrid."

Jim persisted, told his daughter again about his experience in college, about the friends he had made, how he had worked hard but never felt the kind of paralyzing pressure that she seemed to be feeling.

Maddy put down her phone and let her eyes drift toward the window. "You don't know how lucky you are," she said almost wistfully.

"You can have that, too," he said. "I promise."

She shook her head.

"Well, how do you feel about transferring?"

"I don't know," she said. "Vanderbilt could be an option."

Over winter break, she had started looking into Vanderbilt. The school had strong athletics and academics; plus, it was close to Ashley.

In that moment, the word "Vanderbilt" no longer represented a group of distinguished buildings in Nashville, boys in penny loafers and sorority girls drifting from class to class. The school represented something much more elusive: hope. At least Madison was still considering solutions. At least she was still problem solving. This thought soothed Jim.

"Let's plan a visit down there," he said.

"Yeah," Madison replied, noncommittal. "That would be good."

A few minutes later, with Exit 4 fast approaching, Jim turned on his blinker and slowly eased the car off the highway. They cut through New Jersey, past the gas stations and fast-food joints and strip malls, then crossed the Ben Franklin Bridge, and soon enough the ivy-covered buildings of Penn were just outside their windows.

Ingrid Hung was Madison's best friend at Penn. Ingrid's sister Nicole played basketball for Princeton, which is how Ingrid and Maddy had connected, and also why Ingrid had returned early to school. Ingrid was from California, and she and Maddy talked frequently about spending time in Los Angeles that summer. Madison had always wanted to visit the Golden State, so she was thrilled to have a friend from Pasadena, and she sent Ashley a message on Facebook talking about how they should all go west for a week or two in July. Ingrid had come to school in Philly in large part because she had been recruited for the crew team. But now, just like Maddy, Ingrid wanted to quit. She wanted to experience college without the demands of practice and meets.

Freedom. She and Maddy talked about this all the time.

Jim and Madison met Ingrid at Baby Blues BBQ, which was just across the street from Maddy's dorm, between Chestnut Street and Walnut. Inside the quirky space, the first floor of a renovated townhouse, the two friends easily fell back into a rhythm. They'd stayed in touch over break, texting frequently, and even though they'd known each other only a few months, both seemed to believe the relationship would last.

AH you are actually the cutest and best person ever. THANK YOU BEST FRAND!!!!!!!!!! I was going to send ya a long message before your flight left tomorrow but I guess I'll just do it now. Here goes! So in all honesty I don't know what I would have done without you this semester. Even though it took a little time to find each other, and while we are both still in the long and tedious process of finding ourselves (lol will we ever??), I can say that with you here it's made the transition a lot easier. And by no means did I expect the transition to be THIS hard, but each day things are getting better, and I know we will make the most out of second semester and not let the time slip away without loving the rest of our time here. So thank you again for being YOU and becoming one of my best friends. Even though it's only been a couple of months I can confidently say that I hope we stay friends for life. And maybe even pretty soon you can show me some things to do in Cali ☺ 😀. So second semes-ter let's vow to live it up, continue our lunch dates at huntsman, not lose each other when we go out (get leashes), not black out (possible?), sing more karaoke at blarney, get into those damn sororities, and accomplish tasks on our soon-to-be-made bucket list. Also ace that Chinese final tomorrow… REP YOUR RACE!!!!!! Once again thank you and I love ya with all my heart ♥ 👯

At lunch, Maddy seemed to light up around Ingrid, the two of them brainstorming how they would make second semester great. Ingrid brought with her a copy of *The Happiness Project,* the bestselling book about one woman's yearlong pursuit of joy. Jim listened as they talked about rushing for sororities. *How did it work, exactly?* Neither knew for sure, but they cobbled together bits and pieces. They knew the process would start in earnest the following weekend, and they spoke breathlessly about what that might entail.

Jim smiled as he paid the check. Maddy seemed genuinely excited to see Ingrid. And Jim couldn't help but stockpile these moments, these small reassurances that offered him a brief respite from worry.

The Penn-Princeton women's basketball game started at 4 p.m. at the Palestra. They arrived an hour early to watch Princeton warm up—perhaps the only time they would see Jackie in action. Ingrid's sister Nicole was hurt, so she was sitting on the bench in street clothes, and Jackie had missed a few weeks with a broken finger, so she was still working her way into shape.

Nicole had given Ingrid two Princeton practice jerseys, reversible black-and-orange mesh cutoffs that the two Penn friends eagerly put on, Penn's blue and red be damned. That afternoon, their loyalty clearly lay with the Tigers.

Jim, Madison, and Ingrid found Jackie's parents, Susie and Kobus Reyneke, and the group sat in the bleachers behind the Princeton bench, the three adults in one row, Maddy and Ingrid perched just behind them.

Jackie tried to stay focused on the game, but she thrilled at having Maddy in the stands. She was so proud to call her a friend. They had spent so much time in high school talking about this moment, and now here they were supporting each other at college. Even when her eyes should have been on the court, Jackie kept sneaking peeks over her shoulder at her friends and family.

The Reynekes hadn't seen Madison since she'd started college, so during the game they leaned back to make conversation. Madison seemed distracted to them, inside her own head, often staring forward absentmindedly or looking off to the side. She moved around a lot, too, seemed unable to stay seated. Occasionally, when Princeton made a great play, Susie Reyneke would lean back to Maddy and excitedly ask, "Did you see that?" And Madison, having drifted somewhere else, would snap her attention back to the court, saying, "Oh, oh, I wasn't watching—what happened?"

They knew, through Jackie, that Madison was struggling. But many of their daughter's friends were having trouble with the transition to college, exacerbated because most were playing sports and overwhelmed with the time commitment. The truth was, none of the parents had any idea what to say or do—for their own kids, let alone for someone else's.

Of course, the time commitment was just one part of why the transition was so difficult. So, too, was starting again at the bottom of the food chain—and not just any food chain, but a new, more competitive one. Madison, Jackie, Nicole, and Ingrid were going from being the best player on a team, often one of the best teams in the area—sometimes even the state or the country—to being only one among a collection of equally talented athletes. The dramatic shift in status was triggering a crisis of self, since much of a young athlete's ego is fueled by on-field success. Dropped into a situation where positive feedback, that fuel for the ego, was much more difficult to earn, meant that they had to fall back on their still developing sense of self. This was one variable Maddy was dealing with.

"How are things?" Kobus Reyneke asked Maddy during the game.

"Everything is good," she said.

"And how are things going with track?"

"Not that well," she said. "It's tough."

"Well, just hang in there," Kobus said. "Things will get better."

Madison paused, then said: "We'll see."

That afternoon, the Tigers dominated Penn. With about eight minutes left in the game, the coach signaled for Jackie to go in. As she ran to the scorer's table, she glanced again into the stands—Madison was smiling and clapping. Jackie scored the first two baskets of her college career, and the moment seemed perfect because Madison was there to see it, and because Jackie had told her teammates so much about her high school friend. Now they would all get to meet her.

After the game, Jackie quickly showered, then came back out to the court to see everyone. First semester had been challenging for Jackie, too. She was trying to find her place on the team and in the classroom, but this day felt like a promising start to second semester.

"You were amazing!" Madison said, wrapping her friend in a hug.

"I'm so excited you were here," said Jackie. Then she found her parents and hugged them both.

Madison handed her iPhone to the Reynekes and asked if they could take a picture of the three friends in their Princeton gear, with the court in the background. Jackie stood in the middle, hair wet and pulled back, with Madison on her left and Ingrid on her right.

A few minutes later, Madison uploaded the image to Instagram:

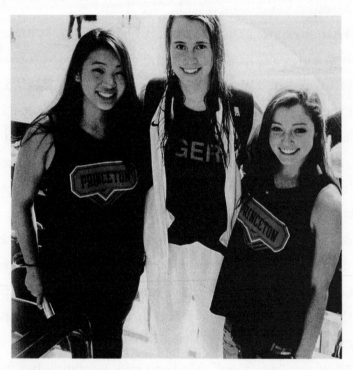

(Madison Holleran Instagram)

Jackie introduced her teammates to Madison, and they all lingered in the stands talking as thousands of fans poured into the Palestra for the men's game, which was also Penn vs. Princeton. The field house, famous for its arched rafters and high windows, is one of the most celebrated college courts in the country, even if it is also a relic compared to the modern arenas in which most Division I teams played. A few of the Princeton women's players were staying to watch the men's game, but Jackie had decided to go back on the team bus.

"Come on," Madison said. "You should stay!"

"I can't, I'm sorry," Jackie said. She would have stayed to spend more time with Maddy, but the two friends had already made plans to see each other: Madison was coming to visit Princeton in just two weeks.

So they hugged and Jackie left to catch the bus. On the drive back to Princeton, Jackie's teammates kept saying how beautiful Maddy was, how striking. Some of them had grown up in the area and knew about Madison because during her high school years her picture seemed to appear daily in the sports section of the *Bergen Record*—first for soccer, then for track. Somehow she always managed to look graceful, her silky dark hair pulled back, often with a red-and-white ribbon, the official colors of Northern Highlands High School.

Jim had to get back to Allendale. Maddy and Ingrid were staying for the men's game, and they invited him to stay and watch with them, but he wanted to get home in time for dinner. Even so, he was reluctant to leave his daughter. He looked at her, noticed again the shifts he couldn't stop seeing: how distracted she seemed to be, the way she wasn't staying focused on anything for long, how her energy was just—off.

She's not happy, he thought. *That's not a happy kid.* But she was with Ingrid, and he knew she adored her friend. And he couldn't stay forever. He couldn't pitch a tent outside her dorm room. She was in college now. Plus, he reminded himself, Stacy and Mackenzie, his wife and youngest daughter, were coming to visit Madison in just a few days. She had a meeting scheduled with the Penn track coach to talk about her future, and they were driving down for moral support.

Jim believed she would be okay until then.

He hugged her, and he thought he noticed that she held on to him for just a split second longer than usual, giving him an extra squeeze before letting go.

"Love you, Daddio," she said.

When Madison got back to her dorm room that night, she sat at her desk and powered up her MacBook Pro. Over winter break, she had asked her friends what she should write to Steve Dolan, the Penn track coach, about how she was feeling. The only problem: none of her friends knew how she was really feeling. Only she did.

She scooted her rolling black chair closer to the desk. Above her right shoulder were four square corkboards onto which she had pinned dozens of photos of her high school friends. One of her favorites was from the New Balance national championships just a few months before. Madison is standing with her relay team, the four of them shoulder to shoulder, beaming.

She began typing.

Although this has been extremely difficult to put into words, I'm going to do my best to explain my first semester at Penn and where it's led me.

Before I begin I just want to say I have the utmost respect and admiration for you as a coach and a person and that I know I wouldn't be at this school if it weren't for you. I also want you to know that you aren't at fault for anything negative I've felt over the past couple months in any way.

Here goes.

In Real Life

I am sitting in the makeup chair inside Media 3, a live-shot studio in New York City just around the corner from Grand Central. The makeup room is small, like a converted broom closet, and in a few minutes I will appear on the ESPN program *Outside the Lines*. The makeup artist is a woman I have known for about a year, although we see each other only occasionally. She has recently had a death in the family, and I ask her how she's doing.

She lowers the brush in her hand, looks directly at me: "It hasn't been easy, but I've realized one thing: being happy is a choice. I have to be strong for everyone around me. And I'm choosing to be happy."

My jaw tightens. I tilt my head. I am not sure if I should respond. She is dealing with a loss, and maybe I should support however she manages to get through her days. And yet, I can't abide the idea she has just introduced into the space between us. Saying nothing feels like tacit agreement, a willingness to perpetuate, even implicitly, this particular idea of happiness as moral superiority.

I open my mouth, then close it, then open it again: "I mean, I hear you, but I'm not sure everyone can choose to be happy. Sometimes whatever is going on in their brain can't just be willed away, you know?"

"You're right, you're right," she says, reaching for the mascara. "But I just think you can't let the demons get you."

"Right, but maybe your demons aren't as persistent as someone else's."

She is mixing two colors of blush and doesn't seem to hear this. After a delay, she says, "Mmmhmm."

I leave a minute later.

I met Megan Armstrong on Twitter. She is a young writer who studied journalism at the University of Missouri, one of the best such programs in the country. We follow each other online. She wrote a novel, and through social media I vaguely gathered that the book touched on issues of mental health and suicide. She also regularly engaged with NFL player Brandon Marshall, an outspoken advocate for mental health awareness. In 2011, the wide receiver was diagnosed with a mood disorder, but rather than hide the news, Marshall publicly announced his diagnosis. He had a platform and had decided to use it to help end the stigma around mental illness. None of the issues that Megan and Brandon were grappling with were in the forefront of my mind.

I am fairly mentally healthy. I mean, I think I am. (Can anyone ever really know for sure?) And no one in my immediate family deals with significant mental health issues. If pressed, I could have offered a general sense of the mental health space, of Megan and Brandon's roles in them, but I had no reason to directly or personally engage with either.

The first time I reached out to Megan, it was because someone who had read Madison's story in *ESPN The Magazine*, in a piece called "Split Image," was direct-messaging me on Twitter, and I felt ill equipped to respond. This person told me they had long battled depression and suicidal thoughts, and that I seemed like someone who was willing to listen. They asked if they could call me. I panicked. I knew very little about communicating with someone who might feel they no longer wanted to live. Megan held my hand as I responded to this reader, making sure they found appropriate help.

Then I started talking to Megan, on text, for long stretches each day, asking her any questions about depression and anxiety that she was willing to answer. Which, as it turns out, was all of them. I had received hundreds of e-mails after Madison's story came out, some more difficult to read than others, one referring to "the monster within."

I wanted to understand, as best I could, what this monster looked and felt like.

May 2015:

> **Kate:** So, it's incredible to me that someone is feeling existence in such a vastly different way.

Megan: I think that all the time.

> **Kate:** I've never been so intensely aware of how lucky I am that, generally speaking, I feel mentally healthy.

Megan: Yes, it's a privilege for sure. I learned long ago that a good day for me is not the same as a good day for most people. Do people such as yourself who are mentally healthy have questions about those who aren't? Because I always have questions about mentally healthy people.

> **Kate:** I have a million questions.

Megan: I'm not an expert, and I don't have letters after my name, but if you ever want to ask them, I'll answer.

Kate: I just wish I could understand. I mean, is my worst day (mentally) better than your best day?

Megan: Probably.

Kate: I'm sure it's all on a sliding scale, and people are in the middle, etc, but if we're just talking someone who doesn't deal with depression talking to someone who does.

Megan: + anxiety + mood disorder. It's quite the cocktail.

Kate: Right. There are a lot of variables.

Megan: But I'm at the point where I can separate my experiences and which of those three — depression, anxiety, mood disorder — caused them, both currently and retrospectively.

Megan: Maddy's experience was mine in very many ways. It was almost spooky. The only difference, of course, is that sadly I'm the only one still here.

Kate: Goodness. So true.

Kate: What do you feel like when you wake up in the morning?

Megan: It usually goes in this order: I spend a minute deciphering whether the dream I just woke up from is reality or not, then I get really pissed that I'm awake, then I lay there for a while scheming ways I can stay in bed for as long as possible and avoid the world. In short: I feel like I've already lost the day just by opening my eyes.

Megan: Oh and then I get sad that I feel that way.

Kate: So the dream is always better than waking up?

Kate: And how do you feel if you wake up in the middle of the night?

Megan: Not always. Sometimes I have really horrible nightmares, which my medications intensify. I also have a photographic memory so it's like impossible to forget my dreams, nightmares or good ones.

Megan: I don't remember the last time I slept the night all the way through.

> **Kate:** When was the last time you woke up in the morning excited for the day?

Megan: Hmmmmmmmm

Megan: No one day stands out specifically in my mind except for Saturday, March 15.

Megan: I don't know if my excited constitutes the same as excited, excited. The night of March 15 was a celebration for a friend of mine who died. Jake is my friend who died from cancer, who I ran a marathon for, etc. So I woke up knowing that I was going to be able to feel him and be with his family that day, so I was more apt to get up and be an active person in life that day. But with that, comes anxiety.

Megan: And the temptation to hide.

Kate: What's anxiety feel like to you? I get anxiety for Around the Horn (not comparing the two, just explaining) and my heart rate is high and I feel slightly panicky and half my brain power is taken up by some bad energy that tells me I'm gonna fuck up. But the more I do it, the less anxiety I feel.

Megan: Anxiety for me feels paralyzing. Horrible word to use, I know, but it's the truth. I'm scared to do pretty much everything. It's like these flurries of irrational thoughts that I know are irrational, but my mind just has them anyway and I can't help but give in to the feeling. Sometimes, I manage it and I go and it's fine. But when it's really bad, I hide.

Megan: In 2013, the summer before my suicide attempt, I lived in Brooklyn with my two cousins and interned with NBC Sports in New York City. It was a night gig. I spent all day binge eating and then I'd be in the bathroom all day just looking at myself and hating myself and hiding from the fact that I had things I wanted to do but couldn't figure out how to do.

Kate: What did you see when you looked at yourself?

Megan: A very fat, worthless, lifeless person who was looking right through herself.

Kate: And what would happen when (if) you tried to tell yourself that wasn't true?

Megan: I would never try to tell myself that. Other people would, and I simply wouldn't believe them. I felt really, really, really embarrassed

and even more of a burden than
before.

> **Kate:** What does being a burden
> feel like?

Megan: I would describe it as really
lonely, but not wanting to be alone,
but feeling like you have to be in this
life alone because dragging anyone
else down with you, especially people you love, is even more selfish
than the thoughts I already have and
things I already did.

> **Kate:** Do you feel like you have to
> pretend to be fine/happy a lot?

Megan: Yes.

> **Kate:** Do you ever wonder why you
> have to deal with this?

Megan: I used to before my friend
died of cancer. Now it's more of,
HOW am I going to deal with this?
WHY CAN'T I figure out how to
deal with this for good? WILL I ever?

Megan: Plus, genetically, I was primed for it.

> **Kate:** How often do you think about this, during the course of a day?

Megan: What qualifies as "this"?

> **Kate:** Mental health. How you'll deal with it.

Megan: Oh, constantly. There are times when I'm doing something and really engaged in the moment but more often than not, during those times, I'm very self-conscious.

Megan: And I worry very much how this will inhibit me in the future. I worry very much, who in God's name will ever want to sign up for this in a relationship? Will anyone want to hire me? Am I really this bad? Am I getting better? What exactly is better?

Megan: And the big one: How honest should I really be?

Megan: The benefits of being honest are great. People come to me when they need help, which is the whole point. I feel like I'm living an honest life. I do wonder if I'm making things worse for myself, but then I remember how miserable I was with this giant boulder in my stomach.

>   **Kate:** Do you mean talking about this so frequently and having people come to you — perhaps that makes you feel it more?

Megan: Nah. I mean worse for myself in terms of alienating myself.

>   **Kate:** Alienating yourself because people will only see you for your issues?

Megan: Correct.

>   **Kate:** (Like in the same way, though not the same, as how I worry people will just see me as the gay one?)

Megan: Yes, like that. We all have our token vulnerability, or what is perceived as vulnerability, and we all work our whole lives to be more than that one token thing.

> **Kate:** While also feeling, sometimes, a responsibility to "normalize" that thing.

> **Kate:** What helps?

Megan: People who care. Doing things I like and feeling rewarded for it. Therapy.

Megan: That might be the toughest question you've asked.

> **Kate:** Why?

Megan: Because I don't know. Everyone wants to feel loved, and everyone wants to feel good at something. But, like, that doesn't make anything go away. I guess what helps is consciously fighting against my own brain. Learning my own brain. Honest conversations.

Megan: Feeling better actually feels worse sometimes because I feel

pressure to never feel bad again,
which is inevitable.

> **Kate:** When you feel better, what
> does that feel like for you?

Megan: Feeling better for me feels
like I can take a deep breath and
not have a daunting thought on the
other side of that breath.

> **Kate:** What does it feel like hoping
> for some better place off in the
> distance?

Megan: That's a complicated, good
question. It gives me a second of
hope and a reason to stay here. But
it also can become discouraging
because I don't get there and I'm a
perfectionist, a destructive perfectionist like Madison. Just like Madison.

> **Kate:** What does it feel like when
> something isn't perfect?

Megan: My therapist tells me, "You
HAVE to remember, you will always
have a distorted view of the world.

Your eyes are skewed. You have a depressed lens. An anxious lens. A perfectionist lens."

Kate: What did reading about Madison make you feel?

Megan: Took me right back, but not in a bad way. I just felt inside her head. I felt like I was reading about me if I had died.

Megan: And it made me glad that people were going to read that and maybe be forced to think for a minute.

Kate: That's surreal.

Megan: I read that quote from Madison's mom, about being so mad at her, and thought about how mad my aunt was when she called me or how mad my mom would have been. She would have been so, so angry at me, because I had promised her I'd never do it back in high school.

Megan: I remember that Saturday, after my attempt, when I woke up at home, my mom was just kind of staring off into space while we were sitting in the living room, and she said, "I don't even know where I would start." I said, "What do you mean?" She said, "Like, you know so many people. Who would I have to call first and what would I even say?"

Megan: I attempted suicide with the intent of dying and relieving my loved ones of me, at least on the surface. But maybe, also, I did it to prove to them, "Look. This is really serious. I'm not bullshitting you."

Kate: Why does therapy help?

Megan: Therapists are magicians. I take that back: GOOD therapists are magicians.

Megan: I learn new coping mechanisms.

Kate: How do you feel about people who don't struggle with their mental health?

Megan: I feel that everyone struggles with their mental health to a degree because life is hard but mental illness is when that struggle inhibits you from your daily life. So, my feeling toward people who don't have that? I'd be lying if I said I wasn't jealous. But I'm not that much of a unicorn. I know people deal with this shit. A lot of people.

Kate: What's your biggest fear?

Megan: Dying before I've had the chance to really live.

Kate: And biggest hope?

Megan: To be able to go day-to-day and feel excited about it — to feel full.

CHAPTER 2

August 23, 2013

Madison woke up early. She sat up in bed, beneath the sloped white ceiling of her childhood room, within its painted red walls. She looked around. Leaning against the wall was the corkboard she would take with her to college, the bib from her national championship race pinned to the top left corner. Across the room was an old white desk on which Maddy had once dangled all the medals she won.

She had been waiting all summer for this day: the day she left for college. Three weeks prior, she had posted a picture on Instagram of one of the most beautiful buildings on Penn's campus, writing, "T–3 weeks left."

Leaving for college was all she and her high school friends talked about. Everything that summer pointed toward the next step. That's how they talked about it, as if that summer was the equivalent of waiting in the boarding area for flights to exotic cities, anticipation clinging to everything. When they were sophomores and juniors at Northern Highlands, a few of their older friends would leave for school, then come home to visit and talk about how they wanted to transfer or take a semester off. Madison and her friends were baffled. They would say, "What? This is so confusing—how can you not like college?"

Madison's sister Ashley was one of these older kids. She would come home every weekend from Penn State and talk about how miserable she was. Madison would press her, confused about what her sister was feeling.

No one among them, parents included, cautioned that the transition to college might be unexpectedly difficult. Part of why no parent did so must have been because they simply could not imagine it would be. College had been different for their generation. For one thing, they grew up without the Internet, without video games, without social media. Madison and her friends were the first generation of "digital natives"—kids who'd never known anything but connectivity. That connection, at its most basic level, meant that instead of calling your parents once a week from the dorm hallway, you could call and text them all day long, even seeking their approval for your most mundane choices, like what to eat at the dining hall. Constant communication may seem reassuring, the closing of physical distance, but it quickly becomes inhibiting. Digital life, and social media at its most complex, is an interweaving of public and private personas, a blending and splintering of identities unlike anything other generations have experienced. Jim and Stacy, Susie and Kobus, and millions of other parents hadn't yet considered how the Internet might be affecting their kids, how it was fostering an increased dependence on outside validation, and consequently a decreased ability to soothe themselves. In 2013, these were just beginning to register as increasing concerns.

When Jim was growing up, good colleges were challenging to get into, but it wasn't like it is today, when being a solid, diligent student is no longer enough. Students today must display excellence—not just competence—in numerous areas. The pressure to be great, not just good, is unrelenting. Believing that this pressure will simply disappear once kids arrive on campus seems like wishful thinking.

In Allendale, college is the ultimate destination, the goal toward which almost every student works. If coming of age used to mean summers and weekends working at 7-Eleven cleaning the Slurpee machine to make a few extra bucks to buy your favorite record, now it's about checking boxes on a college application: becoming fluent in a second language, volunteering at a shelter, taking weekly SAT prep courses.

As move-in day approached, Maddy became anxious about the unknown. But she didn't feel like talking about these feelings. She didn't want to be the one to say, "Hey, you guys, is anyone else maybe a little scared about this?" What if they weren't scared? What if, instead, her friends looked at her, heads tilted, like something was wrong with her?

And anyway, she was mostly excited. She wanted to focus on that.

She got out of bed that morning and waded through her messy bedroom, which looked as if her closet had exploded. Her room was always a disaster, clothes strewn across every available surface—hats and bags layered on hooks, the carpeted floor covered in worn clothes, the dresser with bottles of lotions and perfumes, the yellow chair stacked high with books and notebooks. The space was at complete odds with the rest of her life, which was meticulously presented, nothing out of place.

Maddy had already packed everything that mattered, pre-selecting an outfit for the day: light-blue high-waisted shorts, a pink bralette with a lace shirt, and tan gladiator sandals. And, of course, she wore a running watch on her right wrist so she could time her runs or anything else that needed mea-suring, such as her walk to class or her studying sessions.

Her roommate, Emily Quinn, was also on the Penn track team. The two had met earlier that summer during a team bonding weekend in the Poconos. Maddy wanted to arrive first at the dorm room, mostly because she liked to be first in everything, so she and Stacy left Allendale early.

When mother and daughter walked into the room, Stacy pulled out her iPhone and snapped a candid picture of her daughter. The room is bare, a twin bed on each side, a sallow light glowing from above—it is every dorm room every-where. In the middle of the room, arms raised in a V, stands Madison, palms upward, eyes closed, mouth open in a smile. She's holding a half-eaten red apple in her right hand, and she looks as if she has just stuck the landing on a dismount.

The picture is blurry, but the energy radiating from the image is unmistakable: freedom, euphoria.

Later that afternoon, after all the obligatory errands—to Target, to Office Max, to the Penn student center—Madison was settled in her new space. The bed was made: pink com-forter, accent pillow with lowercase *m*. The desk area was tidy, efficient, colorful, with a pink iPhone dock and pink wastepaper basket, a small black fan on one level, a mug hold-ing pens and pencils on the next. Beneath the desk was a purple plastic container filled with shampoo, body gel, and conditioner. And on the top corner of the tiered desk, angled to lean against the wall, was a piece of art, the background green, with fragments of encouraging sayings. The words, in varying sizes, were stacked like Tetris pieces.

Dream Big
Laugh Out Loud
Be Happy
Just Breathe
Follow Your Heart
Be Grateful

Try
Create Your Own Happiness
Be Silly
Keep Your Promises
Nothing Is Worth More Than This Day

When Stacy and Jim had driven Ashley to Penn State, they had stayed overnight in Happy Valley. Ashley had begged them to. She just didn't feel comfortable. But that afternoon at Penn, Stacy left a few hours after she and Madison had finished unpacking. Maddy was walking to the dining hall for dinner, and Stacy hugged her hard, then got in the car and returned to Allendale. Stacy was not concerned. During high school, Maddy had easily pivoted from one endeavor to the next, smoothly adapting to new sports, to harder classes. Jim and Stacy had always felt that Maddy, self-sufficient and clever, was the child they'd never have to worry about. This next step, to Penn, was harder than anything her daughter had previously faced, but Stacy had only seen her succeed, and believed she would again.

Plus, Penn was only ninety minutes away, not a full day's drive like Penn State, and Maddy seemed excited, ready for the start of this next adventure.

Allendale is a mostly white, upper-middle-class town about twenty miles from New York City. It is farther from New York

City than some of New Jersey's more affluent suburbs, such as Teaneck and Ridgewood and Montclair, which are filled with families whose parents commute daily into Manhattan. Jim travels to the city once or twice a month and spends the rest of his time working from the basement of his home. The Holleran family included five kids: four girls (Carli, Ashley, Madison, and Mackenzie) and one boy (Brendan) who is also the youngest.

The Hollerans live on a street less than a mile from the high school Maddy attended. The road is not a cul-de-sac; it simply stops, becomes woods. Beyond the back of their property, and the soccer goal on which Maddy spent hundreds of hours practicing, is an open field with horses, where kids can learn to ride and jump. The town's personality is flexible, depending on what each inhabitant wants to make of it: some see it as a bedroom community just miles away from the world's busiest city; most see it as self-sustaining, self-contained, thankfully out of earshot of New York's noise and bustle—a quiet haven in which to raise kids.

Northern Highlands High has about 1,300 students. The school also draws kids from surrounding towns, including Ho-Ho-Kus and Saddle River. Even so, Highlands is far from being one of New Jersey's largest high schools.

Allendale's small downtown offers a Starbucks as well as a few local shops, plus a bar and grill where many patrons know one another and where community members often host celebratory dinners. The well-manicured main street is like a slice of Americana, with the Stars and Stripes flying during the height of summer. The town has money: enough that most want for little, but not so much that its residents appear wasteful or excessive, as in some of New York's other suburbs. Like hundreds of other boroughs across the country, Allendale has its distinguishing backstory and quirks: the town was named after William Allen, a surveyor for the Erie Railroad; it is home to the Celery Farm, a nature preserve through which Madison often liked to run; and scenes from the movie *Presumed Innocent,* with Harrison Ford, were filmed there.

Jim and Stacy moved to Allendale when the company for which Jim worked, Dow Chemical, asked him to relocate to the tristate area from Michigan. The move was a welcome one for the couple, as both had grown up on Long Island. The East Coast was more their style, and living there would bring them closer to both their families. Jim and Stacy had actually been high school sweethearts, but their story had a lengthy intermission. The two had known each other since they were little, played tennis together growing up, and dated in high school. But they broke up while in college: Jim at High Point, in North Carolina, and Stacy at Southern Illinois. Each married someone else. Stacy had a daughter, Carli, with her first husband, with whom she lived in Georgia, until the couple divorced. Around the same time Jim, too, divorced. He and his ex-wife did not have children.

Soon the two were back in touch. And not long after that, Stacy and Carli were moving to Michigan to be with Jim, to start a new family together. A few months before their move back east, Ashley was born. Madison was born two years later, on a beautiful, crisp fall day. In fact, the morning of her birth, Jim was at the soccer fields with Ashley, watching Carli play. He remembers the day clearly—how bright and blue the sky was, how he went to the hospital straight from the field, how later that day they added another child to their growing family. Over the next five years, Jim and Stacy would have two more children: Mackenzie, then their only son, Brendan.

Jim continued working for Dow Chemical as an account manager. He had majored in chemistry in college, but now worked in sales. Stacy, who had played tennis in college, began giving lessons, which she still does five days a week.

Jim and Stacy raised the kids as Catholics, but the most religious among them was Jim. As a family, they went to church just a few times a year, always on holidays, and all five kids were baptized and confirmed. Maddy took her confirmation seriously, choosing the confirmation name "Amelia" and later taking the first steps toward exploring her own, independent feelings about God and religion. Still, while in high school Maddy rarely attended church with Jim, who went faithfully, alone, every Sunday morning.

When Maddy was little, her hair was cut short and she loved to play outside. She called those years her "little boy days." When she turned seven years old, she requested that her birthday party feature live animals—snakes and frogs—to be stocked in her family's basement for herself and the neighborhood kids. Maddy loved the outdoors and all its creatures, and probably would have continued having animal parties and running around outdoors getting dirty if the world in which she and other girls live would have approved.

By the time Madison hit middle school, her "little boy days" were a distant memory. She had begun to grow out her hair a couple years before and started caring about how she looked, about the clothes she wore, about what other kids said about her. Still, much of who Maddy was as a little kid had stuck. As a second grader, she had fallen in love with art and soccer. Both helped her make sense of the world. In fact, during her first semester at Penn, Madison took an English class in which she had to give a speech. She started it with an anecdote about soccer: "When you were younger, what did you aspire to be? At some point in our lives, especially as children, we all question what we want to be in the future. In our naïve and hopeful minds, we set big dreams for ourselves. As a third grader I remember setting my goals towards becoming a professional soccer player. During recess I would hop into any pickup soccer games I could; regardless of whether boys were playing or girls. Some of my teammates and I were even invited to play as guests on the boys travel team, and even though they intimidated us a little, we were able to hang in there with them..."

Third Grade

School: Hilbide

Teacher: Mrs. Ebneter

1st Day of School: September 4th 2003

Age: 8 years old

Height:

Weight: 57

Friends: Mary Jane, Remi, Becca, Erin, Sophia, Kaitie, and my WHOLE Soccer team.

Achievements: The American team

Awards: trophies,

Signature: Madison Holleran

School Activities: Gym, Music, Computers, Art

Clubs: Nothing!

Sports: Soccer and Tennis

Important World Events: Playing at half time at Giants Stadium with the Metro stars

What I want to be when I grow up: A pro sports player

(Holleran family)

★ ★ ★

Madison's best friend growing up was MJ White, a friendship forged by the single-mindedness they shared. By second grade, they were playing together on the local club soccer team, forming friendships that would last through high school. And at school, MJ and Madison would spend their free time drawing. One year, they started drawing dogs—different breeds, different names for each. The paper dogs were like pets, but without the hassle and long-term commitment. When they first started, they would look at each other and say, "We have to make them perfect, okay?" And both would nod. Soon after, they were drawing dogs every free moment. Once they built up a collection of a decent size, they decided to sell their paper pets to family and friends. The two friends donated the proceeds to buy hats and gloves for the homeless.

Art became a release for Maddy. During middle school, she would spend her free time sketching. One teacher allowed students to paint different parts of the hallway—creative café, the teacher called it—and Madison would take part every day. Even as she got older and other pursuits became cooler, Maddy continued drawing. She liked that she could control the space. The whiteness of the paper could become anything she wanted—and also only what she wanted. If Madison focused intensely enough, if she was willing to block out distractions, she could produce something flawless.

Soccer wasn't like that. Everything happened in rapid succession, one decision forcing the next. But on the field, a different kind of perfection could be attained. Occasionally a play would unfold with such unexpected rhythm as to feel choreographed, and a kind of beauty existed in that chaos.

For years, Maddy had also played tennis, the family sport. She was good at tennis—really good. So good, in fact, that when she and Jim would attend the U.S. Open, as they did every year, she would watch and wonder if she could some-day play at the highest level. Jim believed she could, of course. He believed she could do anything.

But eventually, around the start of high school, Madison dropped competitive tennis in favor of soccer. When asked why, she said she didn't want to play an individual sport. She spent enough time inside her own head—thoughts bouncing around, sharpening inside her mind—that playing tennis felt too isolating. The sport was as much mental as physical: walking along the baseline after each point, trying to rally if things weren't going well, or to stay grounded if they were. The roller coaster of emotions that was tennis was more than Maddy wanted to handle. Where tennis could trap you inside your own mind, soccer was open, even freeing. And Maddy was also really good at it.

Emma Sullivan and Jackie Reyneke started playing for the local soccer club in kindergarten. Jackie's dad, Kobus, coached the team, called the Americans. When Madison and MJ joined, followed by Brooke Holle, another talented kid from Upper Saddle River, the Americans became a juggernaut. Their reputation grew as one of the most elite local teams in the state. Although most of them could have upgraded to a more prestigious team, the girls continued playing together through eighth grade. They didn't want their time together to end, but they knew that by the time they reached high school they needed to switch teams. They needed bigger tournaments—the kind college recruiters attended—and better competition.

For the girls, leaving the Americans was the end of an era. Madison, Erin, Jackie, Emma, and Brooke were going to high school at Northern Highlands, a public school, while MJ would move to a local private school. They would all stay friends, of course, but Maddy became closer to Emma, Jackie, and Brooke, because they saw one another every day.

The Northern Highlands coaches, teachers, and students all knew of Madison before she started high school. That was partly because of Ashley, who was beginning her junior year, but mostly it was because of how Maddy had distinguished herself athletically, academically, and socially. People saw her as someone with endless promise. She was supposed to make varsity as a freshman, get straight As, and generally rule the school.

The summer before starting high school, Maddy became

anxious. One night, a couple weeks before the first day of freshman year, she and her friend Trisha went over to MJ's house and hung out in the backyard eating ice cream and talking. This was the first time any of Maddy's friends had seen her unsteady, doubting. The transition to high school was the first major challenge for all of them—the first life change they faced with concerns beyond who they might sit next to on the bus. That night at MJ's, Madison had just gotten back from a sleepaway soccer camp at Rutgers, and the first day at Highlands was looming.

Growing up, Madison had spent hundreds of hours, and often well into the evening, kicking the ball into the netting of a floppy white goal that Jim had constructed in their backyard. She studied for tests until she knew every answer. She was doing everything she could, and yet so much still seemed uncontrollable.

"I'm just nervous," Maddy said that night at MJ's.

"About what?"

"What if the older girls don't like me? What if I don't make varsity?" She began crying. MJ and Trisha said all the right things: that she would be great, that everyone would love her, that everything would work out. But their words couldn't make it better. Words meant little. Only excellence helped chip away at self-doubt. And so she excelled.

She didn't make varsity as a freshman, but she was called

up repeatedly and earned important minutes during the playoffs. And by junior year, Madison had become exactly the person everyone anticipated she might. She was a starter on the varsity girls' soccer team, scoring thirty goals that season as Northern Highlands won the state championship. At one point during the title game Maddy had to leave the field with an injury, and everyone held their breath, worried she had blown out her knee. But it was only a tweak and she soon returned to the game, and Highlands won on Maddy's sixteenth birthday.

She started running track during sophomore year, mostly to keep in shape for soccer, but each time she raced, she seemed to get faster. This surprised no one. She was a natural athlete with a beautiful stride, the mechanics already in place — a finely tuned race car that had finally found the track.

In school, she was one of the best students in her class, always sitting in the front row with her notebook open. Her reputation: diligent. While some kids skipped assignments and asked to borrow answers from friends, Maddy did all her own work, always. And when she would walk the halls, the younger girls craved her attention, commenting on her outfit or offering congratulations about the latest game or race, anything to stay in her presence just an extra beat, to absorb whatever flicker of attention she might offer. She would mostly smile and laugh. People liked to be around her because she always seemed to be laughing. And when she wasn't, she made sure she was around friends who could empathize, who understood the anxiety that accompanied ambition.

Maddy was very popular—among both girls and boys. The boys loved the way she looked, but there was also something alluring about the unattainable aura she projected; dating and boys—usually the centerpiece of someone's high school experience—were low on her list. "She had so many other things going on," Emma said. "It wasn't her main focus. Yeah, it was there. She could have pursued a lot of that. But she was so focused on doing well in sports and school. Dating just wasn't her main goal." Throughout high school Maddy casually dated and flirted at parties, but nothing became too serious.

Her commitment to sports eventually paid off. By sophomore year, her first full season on varsity, numerous college soccer coaches had written Maddy expressing interest. And by junior year, dozens of additional programs had her on their radar. She was one of the best players in the state, and had strong academics—a perfect candidate for the Ivy League. Harvard was a possibility. So was Penn. Maddy had been charmed when she and Emma took a visit to Philly during their junior year. She'd fallen in love with the school's proximity to a major city, its beautiful architecture and cachet;

but the Penn soccer coach stopped recruiting her after watching a game in which she played poorly.

A wave of disappointment washed over Maddy, but in its wake came an official scholarship offer from Lehigh. The head coach there, Eric Lambinus, was high on her, believed she could be a great college player. When Lambinus watched Maddy, he saw skill and potential, fueled by her passion for the game. Lehigh had been recruiting Maddy for more than a year and had developed a close connection with her. It was a Division I program and a great liberal arts school. Of course, no college could match the allure and name recognition of the Ivy League. But most of Maddy's friends and family thought Lehigh was the perfect fit for her: she could contribute right away on the field, and the academics would be challenging but not all-consuming.

The Lehigh coaches devoted hundreds of hours to recruiting her. They talked with her on the phone regularly, traveled to watch her games, and hosted her on campus three times. They came to know her as well as any kid they had recruited. And in April of her junior year, Maddy gave Lehigh a verbal commitment, which was essentially a promise that, in November of her senior year, she would sign a national letter of intent to play soccer for them. The "verbal" was not legally binding, but most other coaches stop recruiting a player who has given this commitment. And most coaches did stop recruiting her— at least in the soccer world. The Lehigh coaches were thrilled.

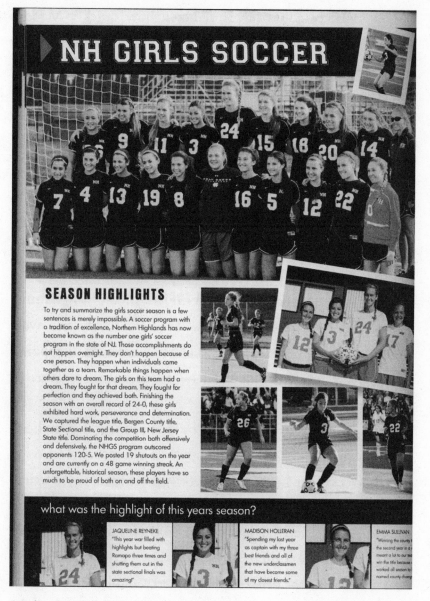

NH GIRLS SOCCER

SEASON HIGHLIGHTS

To try and summarize the girls soccer season is a few sentences is merely impossible. A soccer program with a tradition of excellence, Northern Highlands has now become known as the number one girls' soccer program in the state of NJ. Those accomplishments do not happen overnight. They don't happen because of one person. They happen when individuals come together as a team. Remarkable things happen when others dare to dream. The girls on this team had a dream. They fought for that dream. They fought for perfection and they achieved both. Finishing the season with an overall record of 24-0, these girls exhibited hard work, perseverance and determination. We captured the league title, Bergen County title, State Sectional title, and the Group III, New Jersey State title. Dominating the competition both offensively and defensively, the NHGS program outscored opponents 120-5. We posted 19 shutouts on the year and are currently on a 48 game winning streak. An unforgettable, historical season, these players have so much to be proud of both on and off the field.

what was the highlight of this years season?

JAQUELINE REYNEKE
"This year was filled with highlights but beating Ramapo three times and shutting them out in the state sectional finals was amazing!"

MADISON HOLLERAN
"Spending my last year as captain with my three best friends and all of the new underclassmen that have become some of my closest friends."

EMMA SULLIVAN
"Winning the county the second year in a row meant a lot to our tea win the title because w worked all season to named county champ

Madison (number 3) fell in love with soccer at a young age, and was on the Northern Highlands team that won forty-eight straight games. *(Holleran family)*

But nobody could have predicted how quickly Maddy would improve in track, and by the end of junior year she was posting some of the fastest women's times in New Jersey in the 800 meters. Harvard and Penn were back in the picture. Suddenly, the scholarship offer from Lehigh morphed into a safety net. Maddy needed to see if she could really get into the Ivy League, which was a dream of hers. Or rather, a dream she felt she was supposed to have. Maddy wasn't sure she could tell the difference anymore. She began visiting schools, taking calls, and by fall of senior year, word had gotten back to Lehigh that their prized recruit was wavering.

Eric called Maddy and asked directly if she was visiting schools for their track programs. She said she wasn't even though she was, because she was afraid she would disappoint him. A few weeks later, when he called again, she finally told him.

The Harvard coach said he couldn't support her application, but Penn looked increasingly like a legitimate option, and on December 12, Madison received her acceptance letter. She immediately posted an image of it on Instagram.

On an intellectual level, Eric understood the reversal. Every year he recruited against the Ivy League, and every year his recruits prioritized the name recognition, the prestige. He got that part. He just couldn't make sense of Madison's decision on a human level. She loved soccer: Eric was sure of this. Her passion for the game was what caught his eye from the start. The first game he ever watched her play, he was actually there to scout someone else but fell in love with Maddy. She worked so hard on the field, as if nothing else mattered, which Eric knew meant that the game had worked its way into her blood. Those were the kinds of players he wanted.

Track was supposed to be a complementary pursuit, to help with soccer. She was wildly talented as a runner, but something was missing. Eric had spent hours on the phone with her, mostly in her junior year, and during those calls he had noticed something: a shift in her voice when she talked about possibly running track in college. When she spoke of soccer, her voice was rich, humming with excitement. When she spoke of running, something clinical happened, all hard edges. Running was not creative. Eric believed that her choosing Penn, for track, was a mistake. But it was a mistake he had seen dozens of kids make. During junior year, Maddy had spoken openly with Eric, describing how conflicted she felt about her college decision. *If I get this opportunity with an Ivy, I think I have to take it,* was how Maddy conveyed her thinking to Eric. "But if you don't really want to do it, how can you be successful?" he responded.

The recruiting process seemed to make Maddy uncomfortable: What if what she wanted and what she thought she was supposed to want were opposed? And what if this gap between head and heart happened again? Would she always fall into the space between the two? Penn seemed to offer everything Madison desired: great school, Division I sports, cool city, brand-name recognition. The catch was that to get all that, she had to give up soccer, her first love, the sport that, because of its improvisational nature, forced her out of her own head, forced her to embrace the beauty of the unknown.

Madison officially accepted admission to Penn the month after senior soccer season, the month after Northern Highlands won its second consecutive state title—Maddy and Emma falling asleep on the bus ride home because they were so tired from the game, from chasing that goal.

Excitement about her decision to go to an Ivy League school soon buried whatever inkling of concern Maddy had allowed herself to share with Eric. She was going to be a college athlete at an amazing school. She was becoming the person she had committed to becoming so long ago.

That spring track season seemed to confirm her decision: She was getting faster every time she ran. And she was one of the favorites to win the 800 meters at the New Jersey State Championships, the final meet of the season and the final competitive event of her high school career.

The day of the race, she and Emma sat with each other during the long bus ride. They were both anxious, but Madison especially so because she wasn't a long shot; with one good race, she was likely to become a state champion. She had won two state titles in soccer, but an individual title? That felt different.

Emma remembers the day perfectly: Madison, quiet and introspective before the race, then as soon as the gun went off, sprinting directly for the lead, just going for it, never even looking back.

Emma was standing at the final turn, watching her friend for the final 200 meters. Madison still had the lead. Her face was etched with pain, but Emma noticed that layered above the agony was determination, and she felt that if she were inside her friend's mind at that moment the only thought would be *Get across the line first; get across the line first.*

And Madison did.

In July, Maddy sent an e-mail to local writer Paul Schwartz, who had chronicled her track career at Northern Highlands.

Hi, Paul! Hope your summer is going well! I just wanted to take the time to say thank you for everything you've done for me in track this year. Thank you for nominating me as the Record runner of the year. It was one of the best awards I've ever received... You are amazing at what you do and I'm sure I can speak for all the other runners in Bergen County when I say you are one awesome fan/supporter as well. Thanks again for helping me, nominating me, and supporting me throughout my track career. Hope to see you some-time soon, and if not, I'll definitely be back to watch some meets next year! Have a great rest of the summer.

Madison Holleran

P.S. I will never forget that you told my mom I am like a "horse"…"just keeps going and going." hahaha

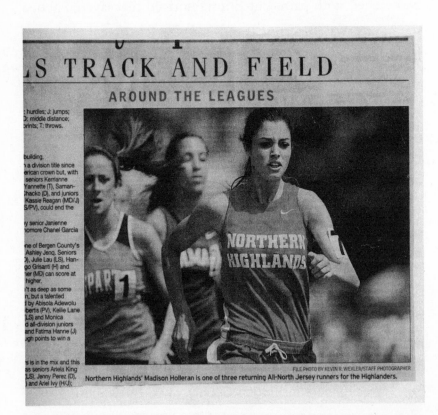

S TRACK AND FIELD
AROUND THE LEAGUES

FILE PHOTO BY KEVIN R. WEXLER/STAFF PHOTOGRAPHER
Northern Highlands' Madison Holleran is one of three returning All-North Jersey runners for the Highlanders.

At first Madison ran track just to stay in shape for soccer, but soon her times were among the best in the state. *(Holleran family)*

CHAPTER 3

The Collapse

The best four years of her life. That's what Madison expected. Four years just like high school, except better—because now she'd be living on her own.

Actually, not quite on her own, living with a roommate. At first, the room she shared with Emily in Hill—the Penn dormitory—seemed just fine, cozy even. For the first few days, they both kept the room meticulous, desperately preserving the image of college life they'd carried around for years: pictures of high school friends above desks, shampoo and conditioner tucked neatly into a plastic carrying case, roommates moving easily around the shared space with laughter and smiles, music blaring, preparing for a big party.

This image soon dissolved. In its place appeared something more real: the messiness and claustrophobia of two people who don't really know each other sharing two hundred square feet, of wet towels left on beds, of books and clothes covering every surface, of neither roommate living up to the expectations of the other, because, well, how could they? This disappointment mattered, of course, but then again so many spaces existed outside that little room in Hill: classrooms, coffee shops, the city, frat parties, restaurants, the track.

... The track.

In high school, track was fun. That was essentially its point: it was a form of cross-training that kept Maddy from burning out on soccer. Track came after school, and she spent much of the time running with Emma, her high school best friend, who competed for Boston College. Pressure eventually arose, once she became one of the best in the state, but she started without any kind of wild expectations. She just enjoyed running. She loved waking up on the weekend and going to the Celery Farm nature preserve, where she could churn through however many miles and whatever thoughts were on her mind.

But track in college was a different beast. For one, it was not just track; it was also cross-country. For another, it was not just one practice after school; it was also scheduled in the morning before classes. It was, like most Division I sports, a job—with time commitments, with demands, with expectations of performance. And nothing turns enjoyment into dread faster than obligation.

Maddy had been recruited to Penn by head coach Steve Dolan. She liked him, clicked with him, and assumed he would coach her. But he didn't. Robin Martin, an assistant coach, was working with her, and the two didn't jibe as well, in large part because they didn't know each other. Thus Maddy was missing a crucial energy source: the inspiration sparked by wanting to make an admired coach proud. At Northern Highlands, she had enjoyed a strong relationship with her soccer and track-and-field coaches. Most high school coaches are also full-time teachers; sports are tangential. And because coaching isn't their livelihood, that layer of stress and urgency, which coaches often pass on to the athlete, is absent.

For all of Madison's life, late summer and fall had meant soccer. It meant walking onto a grass field, cleats in hand, laughing with friends she'd known her entire life. The work was hard, but it was collective work, with friends to connect with between sprints with a nod ("We got this"), or a laugh ("Coach is crazy"), or an exhausted grimace ("How many more?")—each person pulling weight toward a larger goal. Now, late summer and fall meant waking up at dawn in a cramped dormitory room, in a new city, to trudge to practice and run long distances, the person next to you living inside her own head, considering her own times, responsible only for her own motivation. Maddy didn't have anyone she wanted to show up for.

And practices rolled toward her as if on a speeding assembly line, with barely enough time to handle one before the next was upon her, morning then afternoon, morning then afternoon. Emily and Maddy spent numerous moments in their room, looking at each other, wishing they didn't have to leave in just a few minutes to go run — *again*.

Maddy just wasn't enjoying it. The training was so different. In high school, she had been a middle distance runner. She had wanted to stretch to the mile at Penn, but cross-country included races four times that length. Also, when she ran races in high school, she usually won. There were only eight lanes, just seven opponents, but still, Madison routinely finished first. On the other hand, a college cross-country meet included hundreds of runners, all literally corralled at the starting line, released onto the course in a wave of humanity — dense lines of people jostling for running room, fighting to prove themselves with each stride. And each of these runners was just like Maddy: used to winning.

To stay confident, Madison would need a shift in perspective. The same time that had won a race in high school would put her in the middle of the pack in college. But that needed to be okay; she needed to give herself time. Although Dolan thought she was doing well, Maddy couldn't accept the abstract idea that she was doing "well" — not when she had a visceral reminder that she definitely was not. Weren't runners streaming past her on the course?

In early October, Jim went to watch her race cross-country at Lehigh, at the Paul Short Invitational. Penn finished seventeenth as a team, and Maddy came in 104th out of more than 400 runners. That day, she was Penn's second-fastest runner, despite being the only one who hadn't run cross-country in high school. After the race, Maddy introduced her dad to her teammates and the other parents. She was still adjusting, trying to understand if she could work through the pressure and the time commitment. "She wasn't enjoying it like she had in high school," Jim said. "I could tell, but that was a nice little day for the track team, and she had a good race, so that made things better."

On November 2, 2013, Stacy drove to Princeton to see Maddy run at Heptagonals, the Ivy League championships. (Stacy and Jim often alternated who attended what, since of their five kids, three were still playing sports.) Madison didn't say much before the race, because she was too nervous. But Stacy noticed that her daughter seemed different—less radiant, dulled.

The temperature that day was hot, even though it was the first weekend in November, and the course was long, 6,000 meters. Maddy struggled in a way she never had before. She usually had a strong kick on the track and a nonstop motor on the soccer field. She possessed stamina, the result of never cutting corners, of doing all—and often more—of the required work. The way Maddy saw it, people collapsed at the finish line because they hadn't done enough preparation, not because they'd done too much.

But when she crossed the finish that November day, she collapsed. What was happening to her? The medics at the race guided her to the tent, where they checked her pulse, gave her oxygen, and helped her rehydrate. She had finished forty-fourth out of more than one hundred runners, and fifth on the Penn team. Maddy recovered quickly—physically, at least.

Once she was back on her feet, she found her mom and gave her a hug. The color had drained from Maddy's face, but how could it not have? She had literally expended all the energy in her body. "Mom, I'm just not happy," Maddy said that day. "I'm not right—something is not right."

Stacy assured her daughter that it would be okay, that they would figure it out, but she wasn't exactly clear about what was happening. Maddy couldn't articulate precisely what was wrong, only that something was. And Stacy had attended enough of her daughter's games and meets to know how hard Maddy was on herself, how delicate her self-confidence could be.

A few minutes after the race, mother and daughter took a picture together. The moment the iPhone camera turned on, Maddy transformed: she pulled back her slumping shoulders, wrapped Stacy in a hug, and smiled for the camera.

But the reprieve was momentary. And throughout that

fall, Stacy remembers looking at her daughter's Instagram feed and seeing happiness and excitement. "Maddy, you look so happy at this party," she recalls once saying.

"Mom," Madison responded, "it's just a picture."

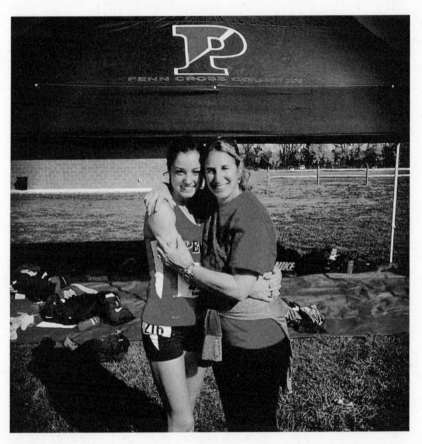

"Post Heps with mama #stacy #Heps #missedya ☺ 🏃." *(Madison Holleran)*

The same night as the race, Madison texted Emma about what had happened.

Madison: THE LEGIT DEATH OF ME

Madison: Never died so hard

Emma: What happened?

Madison: I have no idea

Madison: But I collapsed at the finish line and felt sooooo dizzy I couldn't walk

Emma: Did you do ok?

Madison: Yeah I finished top five on the team so we ended up doing better than we thought we would actually but it was a horrible feeling

Emma: How are you feeling now?

Madison: Much much better. Finally celebrating Halloween!!!!!! We are gonna be party animals

Madison: Ash and I are cheetahs hahaha

Emma told her mom, Lorraine, about Maddy collapsing at the finish line. Emma thought it was unusual, considering how strong her friend usually was in finishing races, but she wasn't tremendously concerned. Madison herself seemed to be downplaying the moment, before pivoting to other matters. But as Emma and Lorraine talked more, really deconstructed what collapsing might mean to Maddy, Lorraine mentioned that of all Emma's friends, Maddy was the least likely to brush off something like this.

Was the collapse only physical? Maddy must be exhausted, but by what, exactly? These questions flashed through Emma's mind, then quickly evaporated. Running was hard. College was hard. Madison would figure it out, just as Emma was trying to do at Boston College. And, anyway, the collapse could be easily explained: hot weather, too little water, too long a distance.

Of course, what remained hard to understand was the effect this would have on Madison's psyche. She had never handled failure, even the garden-variety kind, well. During high school, Madison once finished fourth in the 400 hurdles at a county meet—much worse than expected. She started crying and asked to leave the event, even before cooling down. "She had a tremendous work ethic, and she worked hard at everything she did," Stacy said. "But she just put so much pressure on herself."

In high school, Madison won constantly, and that steady stream of victories strengthened her fragile psyche. But once she was at Penn, Jim and Stacy, along with her older sister Carli, began to notice the erosion of Madison's confidence. When Jim saw her at a meet in October, he told her, "I want to see you in the NCAAs in June."

Madison responded: "Do you really think I'm going to get there?"

Jim didn't miss a beat. "Of course," he said.

"It started to feel like she didn't see herself as a champion anymore," Stacy said. "And she wasn't okay with being good—ever. Good was not good enough."

"I don't think she realized how great she was," Carli said. "Unless she was getting a medal, and then maybe, in that singular moment, she felt it. I would say something like, 'When you're rich and famous, don't forget the little people. I'll be your assistant.'" And Madison would look at her, actually surprised, and say, "What do you mean?" She didn't see what everyone else saw. She was too busy fighting for more, for the next victory, in whatever shape it might come—as small as counting the exact number of steps in a flight of stairs, as big as getting into the Ivy League. For a moment, sometimes longer, these victories slowed the treadmill on which her mind churned, the one that made her feel she could never keep up.

When Maddy was in middle school, she would walk to school in the mornings with kids in the neighborhood. As the year went on, she started timing how long the walk took. Once she had that specific number, she needed the next day to be faster, and the day after that, faster still. By the end of the year, she was speed-walking, occasionally breaking into a jog, to beat the previous day's time. There was something satisfying, calming almost, about controlling time and output in this way. She had created these little tests for herself, ones that she was fairly certain she could pass. That felt good, reassuring: no, nothing was out of her control.

Maddy was addicted to progress, to the idea that her life would move in one vector—always forward, always improving—as opposed to the hills and valleys, the sideways and backward and upside down, that adults eventually learn to accept as more closely resembling reality. Maddy was not unique in feeling this way. Much of young adulthood is presented as a ladder, each rung closer to success, or whatever our society has defined as success. Perhaps climbing the ladder is tiring, but it is not confusing. You are never left wondering if you've made the wrong choice, or expended energy in the wrong direction, because there is only the one rung above you. Get good grades. Get better at your sport. Take the SAT. Do volunteer work. Apply to colleges. Choose a college. But then you get to college, and suddenly you're out of rungs and that ladder has turned into a massive tree with hundreds of sprawling limbs, and progress is no longer a thing you can easily measure, because there are now thousands of paths to millions of destinations. And none are linear.

From second through eighth grade, Kobus Reyneke coached Maddy in soccer. The team practiced three times a week for six years. After a while, he could read her body language, the way her shoulders would sag and her head drop after an imperfect pass or shot. Not necessarily a mistake, just a moment that could have been crisper—the flatness of it often imperceptible to others. When she came over to the sideline, Kobus would stop her, and she would say, "I'm not good."

"Are you crazy?" he would respond. "You're the best on the team!" But no matter how adamantly he reassured her, how vehemently he praised her, this interaction, or some variation thereof, played on a loop for all six years he coached the Americans.

Getting Maddy out of her own head was difficult. She was shy; everyone knew that. But there was a depth to her shyness and the wall she built around herself. She had trouble making eye contact with the parents of her friends. They noticed this when she got into their cars after a practice or a game. The other kids would yank open the door, calling everyone Mr. and Mrs.—all kinetic energy. But Maddy would often keep her head down, her answers monosyllabic. During car rides, she almost always spent the time studying, disconnected from the group. Her friends rarely did homework in the car, but whenever seating became crowded, Madison usually pulled out her books. Not always, of course: sometimes a popular song would come on the radio and she'd start singing and bouncing around just like the rest of them. She liked to smile and laugh, but she also possessed an introspective nature unlike that of the other kids.

At Penn, the chipping away at her confidence wasn't happening only on the track; it was also happening in the classroom. In many of her courses, Maddy was being graded on a curve. She had no experience with curves. She was used to studying for a test, getting most of the answers correct, then seeing a high grade that showed her exactly how she was doing. At Penn, she could study for days, get half the answers correct, and have no clue where that score ranked among those of her classmates. And if she knew only half the answers, wasn't she probably failing?

School had always been straightforward: collect a specific set of numbers and letters, and receive your desired grade. That was not confusing; that was reassuring. Now, she felt as if she'd been dropped onto a course of unknown length without signs or mile markers.

Toward the end of the semester, one of Maddy's high school friends, Justine Moran, drove down to Philly. The two had grown up together. Justine didn't play sports, and because of that, their relationship did not rely on soccer or running as the common thread. When together, the two often gravitated to discussing other topics, which is what they did that day in Philly. Over Greek food, Maddy told Justine how stressed she felt about school.

"I get tests back, and the teacher says, 'Don't worry about this number,'" Madison told her friend. "I have no idea how I'm doing. I think I'm failing." Justine did her best to reassure Madison that everything was fine, that she was going to be fine. After all, hadn't Madison always performed well, even when things became difficult? Why would this time be any different? "I just feel like I'm trying so hard and nothing is working," Maddy said.

Justine could sense her friend's unease. "In high school, she had the perfect—well, everything," Justine said. "She always stood out. But now, she wasn't fully seeing her success, or all of her work paying off. She didn't stand out there as much as she did at home. She was just another person, and it felt like that was scaring her."

Maddy often expected the worst. To her, the prospect of failing out of Penn did not feel like hyperbole; it felt like the probable outcome. How could she believe otherwise, when she had no concrete evidence to the contrary? Everything had been flipped on its head, had become abstract. She was finishing behind a hundred other runners and was told that was good. She knew only half the answers on an art history test and was told not to panic.

Freshman year of college, especially for those playing a

sport, is like walking through an obstacle course wearing a blindfold. No context exists for how hard the workouts will be, how long they will last, what each class will be like, what events are fun, what should be avoided. There is no yin-yang, either; no understanding that one week might feel grueling, unmanageable, but just hang on, because the following week will be light and easy. For someone who struggles with the unknown, freshman year of college can feel like walking a path lined with land mines—heart racing, disaster around every corner.

Now add another variable: mental health.

Mind, Body, Spirit

In the early 2000s, I played college basketball at the University of Colorado. A month into my freshman year at CU, I began to dread practice. This is not an exaggeration; I once swallowed an entire bottle of iron pills in the hopes that I would become violently ill so I could be excused from that afternoon's session. Apparently, I believed that spending hours hunched over a toilet was more pleasant than being on the court. Every single day was the equivalent of me holding a thermometer next to a lightbulb, desperately trying to convince someone, anyone, not to make me go. I found myself focusing on whatever small aches and pains I had. A bruise on my shin was likely shin splints, a sore knee tendinitis. And if I complained persuasively enough, perhaps our trainer would tell me I needed to take a few days off.

The hours before practice became a mental battle far more torturous than whatever I was hoping to avoid on the court. Anxiety dimmed my every waking moment. (And often my sleeping ones, too.) Every minute was one minute closer to the next practice, even if it was just one minute removed from the last. I convinced myself I hated basketball. Then this thought would send me spiraling: Who was I if not an athlete? I didn't know. My identity was as a basketball player. The initial fatigue was, at a base level, physical: difficult morning workouts, increased weights in the gym. But previously, physical strain had always been manageable. I'd always had a comfortable emotional foundation. My feet were planted. A workout was challenging, but it existed within my routine: I went home to my bed, in my room, with my family. Once the foundation shifted, and once my support system became a group of people less warm and caring than my parents, every physical act seemed more difficult.

After about three weeks of this, I walked into the office of Kristen Payne, our athletic trainer, sat in the chair opposite her desk, and started crying. I was lucky. We had developed a close relationship from my first day on campus; I trusted her. As I sat crying in her office, she defended me, dismissing each coach who came into the training room looking for me, wondering why I wasn't yet on the court.

"She's not practicing today," Kristen said.

"But why not? Is she hurt?"

"She's just not practicing today. End of story."

That day, she connected me with a counselor, one not affiliated with the school. And once a week for about a month,

I drove the few miles to his house outside of Boulder, to talk to him and try to unravel what was happening.

I was embarrassed about having to see someone. I told no one I was doing this. I felt weak. The saving grace was that I was spared the discomfort—unfortunately, that's how it would have felt to me then—of walking across campus and into the building that housed counseling services. Everything I did, except for attending classes, was within the silo of the athletic department: lift, practice, study, train, eat—even worship. This was my safe space, my comfort zone. And guess what? There was no counseling center, no psychologist's office, within the athletic department building. The clear message: needing a psychologist is abnormal.

How could an athlete with a mental health issue not feel like an outsider when she was literally forced out of the athletic department and pointed toward a building far away from campus and the athletic bubble? But regardless of distance, therapy helped me; things gradually started to feel better. And within a month or two, I could step onto the court without panicking.

My sister, Ryan, ran cross-country and track at Dartmouth during the same years I played at CU. She was often hurt during college, and in the fall of her senior year, her times plummeted. She just could not get her body to do what her heart and mind asked of it. After one meet—it might have been after Heptagonals, the same race after which Maddy collapsed—my parents found her by herself, crying. Nothing they said could make it better.

Parents don't really know how to help. Some aren't prepared for this new version of their high-achieving kid: doubting, sad, tired, confused—emotions they may have rarely dealt with in high school. And isn't college supposed to be even better than high school? When your child is more mature, self-sufficient, and otherwise flourishing just as she always has been, except now at an even higher level?

The relatively early age—sometimes as early as elementary school—at which parents define children as athletes makes it more difficult to cultivate other parts of their identity. Very little else in our society is rewarded as athletics are. And when you're young, the distinction between an activity that truly satisfies your soul and one that merely brings accolades is difficult to parse. For many, those two things aren't mutually exclusive. For others, sports are actually not their passion, a realization that doesn't come until they're put into the fire of college sports. But admitting ambivalence of this kind can feel like considering filing for divorce the day after a wedding: everyone involved has already invested so much time and money. And hadn't you convinced yourself you were truly in love?

Ryan was eventually found to have anemia, a diagnosis that took far too long to reach, and she immediately began taking iron. By track season, her times dramatically improved.

But for those few months when her body was playing tricks on her mind, which led to her mind playing tricks on itself, she was nearly inconsolable, and it became clear how much self-worth we both had wrapped up in being high-achieving athletes.

Anemia has nothing on mental illness, although with both, people often assume you're just weak and can't push through. We have little sympathy for injuries that we can't see and touch, for whatever is hurting that isn't bloody or outwardly broken. But that's where the comparison between the two ends, because with mental illness, unlike anemia, an official diagnosis usually doesn't end the stigma. And to make matters worse, those with the least empathy are often teammates—peers.

In the spring of 2016, I spent a week at the University of Oregon talking to student-athletes. One evening, I spoke about mental health with the Student Athlete Advisory Committee, and the first question directed at me was, "How can we think differently as athletes, because from the first day we step on campus, we're taught that champions never quit and perseverance is what makes greatness? I'm worried a teammate might be really hurting and all I see is weakness."

No good answer exists for this question, which was the response I gave. I told this young woman that I could deliver the most beautiful monologue about compassion and understanding, but no young person has been compelled toward empathy just because someone implored them to be. I then shared my own personal experience: I was too harsh on teammates who, for example, had transferred (we labeled them "traitors"); only years later did I come to see that just because a situation was right for me didn't mean that it was right for everyone, and sometimes making a life change is fundamentally necessary for another person. Achieving that kind of insight took almost a decade. And what good did it do those scorned teammates I no longer spoke to? Perhaps the only relevant advice I could offer the Oregon athletes was this: Recognize that empathy might be in short supply. Educate yourself about mental health. And consider the idea that not every struggling teammate is weak.

I had this discussion with student-athletes, but the sentiment could have applied to much of the campus population. According to pretty much every study conducted over the past five years, levels of empathy among college-age students is plummeting. The University of Michigan conducted a study in 2014 that found that college kids are 40 percent less empathetic than they were just twenty years before. Researchers at Michigan's Institute for Social Research shared their thoughts on why: "The ease of having 'friends' online might make people more likely to just tune out when they don't feel like responding to others' problems, a behavior that could carry over offline. Add in the hypercompetitive atmosphere and inflated expectations of success, born of celebrity 'reality shows,' and you have a social environment that works against slowing down and listening to someone who needs a bit of sympathy."

After I spoke at the University of Oregon, a young woman approached me and shared the following: "Thanks for talking about empathy. Hopefully my teammates were listening. Sometimes it seems like it's hard for them to focus on anything other than winning. And so then anyone going through something that remotely compromises that pursuit, like I am right now, gets ostracized. I feel like they talk about me behind my back instead of trying to understand."

When it comes to mental health among athletes, clinical diagnoses are rare. Truth is, it's unusual for an athlete to be open and honest with a coach or trainer. I was lucky that I had connected with our team's trainer before my anxiety struck. She knew me on a few different levels: as an athlete, as a student, as someone who enjoyed talking about books, as an eighteen-year-old kid from New York. On some level, I think I understood that even though I felt I was failing at one identity—athlete—she saw my value on other levels and would recognize that I was more than someone who just happened to put on a Colorado jersey. And I needed her to validate my other layers of self-worth, the kind independent of basketball, because I was not yet capable.

During those months at CU, I thought I was alone, the

only student-athlete who couldn't deal with the transition to college, couldn't deal with the time commitment, the added pressure, the morphing of my sport from something I loved into something I loathed. Everyone was strong. I was weak. Everyone was succeeding. I was failing. Why would I think otherwise? All the signals I had ever received indicated that I was the lucky one. I was living a dream. Being a big-time college athlete? I should relish that—love every minute. So what was wrong with me?

Nothing, actually—turns out I was in good company. In 2014, the American College Health Association surveyed nearly twenty thousand student-athletes. Some 28 percent of female student-athletes and 21 percent of males reported feeling depressed, while 48 percent of female student-athletes and 31 percent of males reported feeling anxious. Approximately 14 percent said they had seriously considered suicide, with 6 percent saying they had attempted it.

Of course, it's safe to acknowledge feelings of anxiety and depression, even suicidal thoughts, in a survey. A survey is anonymous. Actually telling a coach or trainer about those feelings is another matter entirely. And even more unusual is the coach or trainer who knows precisely what to do.

Talking openly about debilitating thoughts and emotions might seem like a logical and necessary step for an athlete, until you consider that sports are built on the pillars of tough-ness and perseverance. Picture every Hollywood sports movie, ever. One thing they all have in common: a montage of the lead character pushing through the pain, training to become the best. Our culture celebrates harder, faster, stronger. Vulnerability, it would seem, undermines that pursuit. And within sports culture, continuing to practice or play, no matter what your mind or body says, is romanticized: T-shirts are emblazoned with quotes, inspirational sayings are stenciled on the locker room wall, epic speeches are given. At Colorado, a saying above one doorway read "Pain is weakness leaving the body."

Imagine, with that sign hanging over you, telling a coach you can't run that day. Not because your body hurts (and what kind of hurt is bad enough?), but because your brain does. Many coaches believe these moments are forks in the road, and that choosing to push through pain—in whatever form that pain comes—is what creates champions. Athletes often believe this, too. And it's not entirely wrong. Pushing through pain, clearing hurdles others have crashed into, is how an athlete improves. Knowing the difference between a hurdle and a brick wall is also crucial—yet recognizing that difference is almost impossible when you're eighteen years old. That's the coach's job. And if a coach isn't sensitive to brick walls, athletes are often left to engage in debilitating mental warfare: one part of the mind says *no more;* the other part tells them they're weak for saying *no more.*

The National Collegiate Athletic Association has recognized

how much work must be done to address the mental and emotional well-being of student-athletes, and also admits that for too long, it's been a vastly less significant priority than promoting their physical health. If the variance in spending weren't so disconcerting, the difference would be laughable. Consider the state-of-the-art equipment, expansive weight rooms, training rooms, and practice fields at most Division I schools. If a football player pulls a hamstring, nearly half a dozen licensed professionals hover over him, discussing the most innovative ways to rehabilitate his strained muscle. Yet if most athletic departments' commitment to mental and emotional health were visualized as a weight room, it would more closely resemble this: a few rusted dumbbells, a cracked mirror, cobwebs, and plenty of open space waiting to be filled.

These are the conditions in which many student-athletes train and play. Getting better in such circumstances is almost completely up to the individual.

In 2014, the NCAA deemed the issue of mental health so pressing that it commissioned a paper on the topic that included stories from former athletes, data, and best practices. "In sports like football, toughness is celebrated and weakness is despised," writes former National Football League lineman Aaron Taylor in this paper. "We do what's necessary to navigate this 'manly' environment, and that means masking our feelings. Players learn to 'suck it up,' 'rub some dirt on it' and 'gut it out,' usually with positive results. We're so conditioned to do this that we often default to such behavior in our everyday lives. Unfortunately, masking emotional issues doesn't work as well in the game of life as it does helping us play through a high ankle sprain. It also helps explain why so many emotional and mental health problems go unnoticed. Players become masters at keeping their game faces on all the time, often until it's too late."

According to the NCAA, suicide ranks as the third most frequent cause of death among student-athletes—behind accidents and cardiac failure. Colleges and universities do have policies and procedures in place to respond to a student-athlete's mental health issues. The concern is that the quality of the response, and the intrinsic understanding of the issues, is often subpar, especially when compared to everything we know and study, and discuss at length, about an athlete's body.

Athletic departments more often than not have numerous staff members fully certified to treat physical injuries, yet most don't have a single licensed mental health professional on the full-time payroll. For some departments, this isn't a conscious omission; they've simply never considered the necessity. For others, it's about cost, about where their money will have the most impact. And quantifying the productivity of a training staff—in ankles taped and injuries rehabbed—is much easier than gauging that of a mental health professional.

According to a 2014 article on ESPN, fewer than twenty-five Division I athletic departments employed a psychologist on staff. The importance of a psychologist is this: she may be the only staff member whose job is not related to winning. Even the most compassionate coaches and trainers are dependent on the physical performance of their athletes. It's a nice bonus if they graduate healthy human beings, but that's not specifically why they're drawing a paycheck.

The NCAA is playing catch-up, trying to patch the holes. "One in every four or five young adults has mental health issues," Timothy Neal, assistant athletics director for sports medicine at Syracuse University, told ESPN. "But what is unique about the student-athlete is they have stressors and expectations of them unlike the other students that could either trigger a psychological concern or exacerbate an existing mental health issue."

Some of the stressors and expectations are tangible; others are not. Though it defies logic, many young athletes, on signing a college letter of intent, convince themselves that the hardest work is behind them. They understand there will be practices and training once they get to campus, but this may be seen as maintenance. The toughest work—the development of skill through thousands of hours of practice—has already been completed. Now it's payoff time, an opportunity to be celebrated on a bigger stage. Also, most college scholarships (of the nonathletic kind) reward prior achievement; once a student arrives on campus, there are no daily expectations, though many academic scholarships do require the maintenance of a specified grade-point level. The time commitment for a student-athlete often ranges to twenty-five-plus hours a week. And it's grueling, exhausting work that tests your character and resilience during a time—freshman year of college—when those attributes are often at their lowest levels.

Until recently, the majority of athletic departments weren't proactive or preventive; they simply reacted as best they could if an athlete had a mental health issue. Now some schools are trying to equip kids with the tools to strengthen their minds, to handle their emotions. At Texas Christian University, the athletic department administers a mental health baseline assessment for each athlete before the beginning of the season. A number of universities are doing the same. This way, if an athlete's behavior changes, the trainer has a way of evaluating whether it's significantly different than it used to be. "Most of college athletics is: 'Can he run, can he jump, can he shoot?'" says TCU athletic director Chris Del Conte. "And the whole part of the kid is lost. What do you do with the whole of the kid, with those with eating disorders, with the cutters? It's amazing that coaches are not prepared to deal with this stuff. So a lot of times you have to help them help themselves. 'Let me take this off your hands,' or, 'This is how you have to deal with this. I know performance is the greatest thing you're looking for, but here's what we need to do to get there.' Some of our coaches get it already. Other coaches, it's foreign to them."

Molly McNamara ran cross-country and track for Stanford while also struggling with depression. She wrote a piece for the NCAA touching on issues of perfection, injury, toughness, depression, and empathy. At first Molly felt she was unique in her struggle, until she looked around and realized that a number of other athletes at Stanford were dealing with stressors—all coping in various ways. She told herself, "I am not imagining this...this is actually a big issue." And as Molly recognized, runners, like Madison, often battled their minds in a distinctive way:

"How do you survive those less-than-perfect situations when discipline isn't enough? When grittiness gets you through the workouts but can't seem to get you through the rest of the day? As a runner, you're highly in tune with your body, and you know its highs and lows; you know your normal aches and pains, and you know when you should probably see the athletic trainer. Learning the highs and lows of your mind is much harder."

CHAPTER 4

Vacuum

When Ashley was a student at Penn State, she was unhappy, out of place—a feeling that started the day she arrived on campus. During her first semester, she would spend the weekdays at school trying as best she could to make it work, then right after her final class on Friday, she would drive home to Allendale—three and a half hours each way. Once she turned onto her street and walked in the door of the house, she felt like her old self again—happy, carefree, stable.

Maddy was a junior in high school then, Mackenzie a freshman. Maddy could not comprehend that Ashley did not love college. Even though nothing Ashley said could make her understand, Maddy still pressed her, asking questions as if her older sister's life was a social science experiment.

"So, just to clarify, you're telling me you don't like college," Maddy said.

"Yes."

"Huh," said Maddy.

Of course, once Madison was a few months into her own freshman year, she started asking Ashley different questions about how she had felt at Penn State, and, more important, how she had felt when she wasn't at Penn State.

"Tell me again: What was it like when you were at school?" Maddy asked.

"I was just unhappy; I didn't feel like myself."

"Okay, and how did you feel when you came home?"

"Happy—like myself again."

Maddy looked down. "Oh," she whispered.

Madison was trying to decide whether transferring was the solution. Everyone in her immediate family seemed to believe she just needed to leave Penn. They had all come up with the same superficial solution: a change of scenery, trading the inner-city vibe of Penn for something more laid-back, maybe in the South. Maddy went back and forth. She was texting all her high school friends, even the ones she wasn't that close to, about how much she hated Penn. Yet when Maddy heard that Jim was telling his buddies she wasn't enjoying school, she went to Stacy and said, "Please tell Dad not to do that."

Maddy seemed intent on controlling her own message, even if she had a tenuous grip on what that message was. Part of her wanted to believe the solution was as simple as transferring, but when she tested that logic with Ashley, she found it wanting.

"And how do you feel when you're at school?" Ashley would ask Maddy.

"I hate it."

"Okay, but then when you come home, how do you feel?"

"I'm still unhappy," Madison would say. "Nothing seems to make it better."

"That's just not how I felt at Penn State. I knew the problem was with the school, because the second I left campus, I was happy again."

"I'm not happy anywhere."

"That's different."

"Yeah, it is."

Maddy didn't want to leave Penn since she knew the unhappiness was not simply environmental. She knew that whatever she was suffering from was being carried inside her. Escaping it—escaping herself—was impossible; everywhere she went, the unhappiness came, too. What if she did trick herself into believing a different set of buildings and new logo would fix what was happening? What if she did transfer, but then nothing changed? What if she was walking around that new school, the pain as sharp as ever? That would be scarier than never leaving Penn at all. Living with a ghost is frightening enough, but if you change houses to escape it and the ghost is present in the new space, then you've confirmed that it's not the house the ghost is haunting. It's you.

But neither could Maddy dismiss transferring. Maybe, she kept telling herself, she had it wrong; maybe transferring would be just the thing, despite evidence to the contrary. Maddy wasn't sure how to make herself feel better. She knew what used to make her happy: a finely tuned balance of sports, school, and friends. In high school she was a champ at all three, and each fueled the others. After a night of partying, she liked getting up to run, to sweat out the alcohol; then that afternoon she'd spend a few hours studying, decompressing. Each part was connected to the next, like a spiral staircase that seemed to lead always higher. In high school she even had time for herself, to draw and read, to write down quotes, to be inside her own head without an agenda.

This is what she wanted at Penn, and Madison continued to try to find each part and connect them. But instead of everything building toward something better, something more whole, it felt like everything was unraveling. She would get up early for morning practice only to arrive at classes feeling zapped of energy, which caused her anxiety about how she would make it through afternoon practice. At afternoon practice, she would stress about what she might have missed in class because she was tired, and by the time the day's obligations were over, she had little energy left to go out and develop the kind of natural, easy friendships she'd had in high school.

At first she convinced herself the problem was time management—specifically, her own sloppy time management. Madison believed she just had to plan better. If she wanted to be happy, she would need to be more diligent about her pursuit of it. So she started blocking off time on her schedule for each endeavor. Of course, happiness is often most elusive to those actively chasing it, but that didn't stop Maddy from trying. She and Ingrid would often have sessions when Maddy clearly explained the objectives of each part of the day: practices, classes, studying, socializing. The whole thing felt color-coded, like blocks of time on a child's calendar. Routine had always comforted her. Perhaps now it would save her.

Everything was in her control, except the one thing that wasn't: this pain that had embedded itself inside her, somewhere she could not find, and no matter how tightly she controlled everything else, it wouldn't go away. Where she may have exerted the most control was in her social accounts—her favorite being Instagram. Unforeseen variables consistently affected her daily game plan, her life at Penn, but she had end-to-end control over the images that told the story of her life. Even if Madison was not having the college experience everyone told her she should be having, she could certainly make it seem like she was.

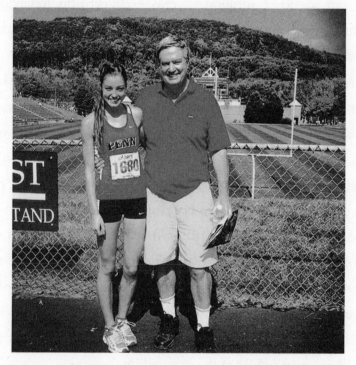

"Love when Ma Jimbo comes to watch." *(Madison Holleran)*

In life, counterintuitive correlations exist between a number of behaviors: we often assume that those who speak highly of themselves do so because they possess a wealth of self-confidence. Of course, bragging is often just a hollow stand-in, a kind of scarecrow meant to distract from the gnawing reality of insecurity. We often label someone who loves going out dancing and drinking a free spirit, when often they're trying to escape feeling trapped. Things are rarely as they seem, especially if overcompensation distorts the image we're presented. This is also true for Instagram: the more polished and put-together someone seems—everything lovely and beautiful and just as it should be—perhaps the more likely something vital is falling apart just offscreen.

At Penn, Maddy used to work out with her friend Ashley Montgomery, who also ran track for the Quakers. On off days, they would go to the gym together or go running outside. Once, in mid-November, the two of them went for a run through the Penn campus. Madison spotted a quote, part of a mural, on the side of a building. She asked Ashley if she could stop and take a picture, which she uploaded to Instagram. A minute later, the two continued running. A few hours afterward, when Ashley went to Instagram to see the picture, the image was gone. Madison had deleted it. This happened another time, too, with another quote; this one Madison uploaded from the gym while they were both working out.

What exactly was the correlation between the two deleted posts, Ashley can't say for certain. Maybe the quotes were too negative, too preachy; or maybe they too accurately reflected an internal struggle Madison quickly realized she didn't want others to see. Then again, maybe it was nothing of the kind; maybe she just didn't like the look of the pictures—they didn't measure up. Something may have felt off about them, and that she could not abide.

★ ★ ★

As November wore on, Maddy became increasingly anxious and uneasy, but her family and friends weren't raising a red flag. They were aware—how could they not be?—that freshman year at Penn was not going as Maddy had expected and that she was struggling with that reality. She texted her parents frequently—or rather, her parents texted her and she responded. But she didn't call them multiple times a day, as did some of her classmates.

Her life had always gone as Maddy expected it would go, as she predicted and willed, despite her near-constant worrying that it would not. Perhaps, her parents thought, she had started to believe that that's how life worked. There was a sense in her family that maybe Maddy would learn a crucial life lesson: how to navigate life when it didn't seem to yield.

Also, the Hollerans had four other kids to worry about. Carli was married, and she and her husband, Scott, were expecting their first child, a boy, in just a few weeks. Ashley was now happily settled at the University of Alabama, which she loved. And Mackenzie and Brendan were both at Northern Highlands, where each played several sports and did everything else young teenagers do.

Maddy was, of course, a priority, but there was no shortage of kids to check in on, to keep safe. Stacy and Jim knew that their middle daughter needed help, but they figured they would work with Madison over the coming months to try to understand what might make her happy. When it came to Madison's troubles, they both felt they had one commodity in abundance: time.

By Thanksgiving break, Maddy's anxiety and unease were morphing into something she couldn't name, and she was visibly struggling to stay present in the moment. Jim and Ashley, who had flown home from Alabama, drove to Philadelphia on Tuesday to pick her up for the holiday. She didn't have to return to Philly until Sunday, yet from the moment she sat down in the car, Madison was already projecting five days into the future and anticipating the sadness that returning to campus would bring. "This week is going to go too quickly," she told her dad before it had even begun.

Maddy was trying to solve the problem on her own. She had always been an incongruous blend of independence and dependence, which most of her friends and family actually found quite charming. She never leaned on anyone else for her homework, and she self-motivated with nearly everything she did. And yet she never got her driver's license. Almost every other kid in Allendale was at the DMV on their sixteenth birthday, but Maddy let that day come and go—then every day after it. She didn't think she would be very good at driving, and the way she saw it, failing the driving test would be worse than never taking it. But also, she just didn't see the need. All her friends could drive. She never found herself stranded anywhere, wishing she could drive, and she liked how it connected their group—everyone always planning who would pick up whom and when.

In mid-November, Maddy decided to make a counseling appointment with Penn's Counseling and Psychological Services. She did not tell her high school friends, or her parents, that she was reaching out to get help. She sat with her Mac-Book Pro and researched the protocol for setting up an appointment, and quickly discovered that the first step was booking an initial screening, a session in which she would talk with someone about what was bothering her so the counselor could assess what kind of help she needed. Maddy had assumed she could see someone the next day, or at least that same week, but in fact the first opening in the system was approximately two weeks away. If her symptoms were time sensitive, if she were desperate, she could have skipped places in the line, but she was not sure she qualified. Maddy accepted the standard initial appointment, waited her turn, and continued trying to fight through whatever this was.

When the date finally came, she was actually hopeful, filled with a belief that the therapist might know exactly how to help, some special trick in the way a physical therapist can soothe a sore muscle or a coach can find just the right game plan. Maybe, Maddy thought, an outsider could see an angle she had missed. No, obviously the therapist couldn't fix everything, but perhaps she could set her on a course toward full health.

The meeting was nothing like what she'd hoped. She felt the therapist had standard questions she asked of every student who walked into the office, and none of them seemed to get at the gravity, the depth, of Madison's situation. *Have you ever been homesick before? How many times a day do you call your parents? Are you making sure you're eating three meals a day?* The meeting, she would tell her family over Thanksgiving, seemed pointless. She understood that homesickness and stress were common issues among college freshmen, but she could not reconcile that those were her issues, because how she felt did not feel common at all. The way Madison felt was extraordinary—and not in a good way.

She tried to convey this to her family over Thanksgiving. She was much better at expressing her feelings in writing, always had been. But that week, she tried to make them understand that something significant was going on.

They started to get it.

Madison was focused and diligent, but in high school she had also been silly and goofy. She was usually smiling, loved dancing and singing in the car when she was with her friends, and also making silly faces for Snapchat. She would often retreat into herself when parents were around. But when it was just her friends, she was usually open and connected. That version of Maddy was not the one who showed up for Thanksgiving. At some point during that week, while the family was in the living room watching one of their shows and the rest of the kids were joking and laughing, Madison was simply sitting there, staring at the screen but not really watching.

"You never smile anymore," Brendan finally said, more as observation than criticism. "You never laugh anymore."

Madison just nodded.

Theirs wasn't the kind of house in which you could hide how you were feeling or what you were doing. It was a cozy little two-story home at the end of a dead-end road, and if you were singing in the shower upstairs, everyone would hear. The place was bursting at the seams—especially during the holidays, when all the kids were home.

Madison sat at the table with Carli and Scott after Thanksgiving dinner. The long wooden table occupied almost the entire space of the eat-in kitchen, with the wall-length window looking out onto the backyard, the soccer goal, and the horse pasture beyond. Maddy had spent hundreds of mornings at that table, eating cereal or peanut butter and bananas. And she had spent countless evenings there studying, eventually closing her books to join Mackenzie just a few yards away, where they would watch *The Voice* or *American Idol.*

That afternoon, the three of them began talking. Carli, like the rest of the family, was not overly concerned, and felt this challenge, a little bit of turmoil, could be good for her sister. "This is normal," Carli told her younger sister. "People leave home, they're unhappy, they transfer—they figure it out." Madison shook her head: "It's not normal. It's not normal to feel like this."

To some degree, Maddy had an easier time showing her vulnerability to her family than to her friends. Still, opening up was not, in general, a comfortable state for her—or, really, for any teenager. Those years are often spent pretending you've developed a tough exterior, because you think you're expected to have one and because you haven't yet realized that a tough exterior isn't actually an asset. Maddy thought being a college student was synonymous with being an adult, which somehow was supposed to be synonymous with individual problem solving—a mistake we all make and most of us recover from.

All of Maddy's high school friends were home for the holiday. Emma was back from Boston College for a few days, Jackie from Princeton, Justine Moran from Marquette, MJ White from Villanova, Brooke Holle from Holy Cross. Except for Brooke, who had fallen in love with her school and team right away, the common theme among them was disappointment and melancholy. College was not as expected. Jackie even told Maddy that she had seen a therapist at Princeton, which empowered Maddy to tell Jackie that she had done the same at Penn but that she hadn't connected with the counselor.

Each of them took turns sharing their own stories from the first three months of school, with most of them touching on the same overarching theme: *Ugh, this is hard; I hope it gets better.* Within that context, nothing Maddy shared over Thanksgiving about how she was feeling drastically separated her from the group. They all knew she was struggling; but so were they, and when you're stuck in the valley, it's difficult to see that perhaps some peaks are sharper, higher, and more dangerous than others. In fact, when you're in the valley, it's difficult to look up at all. Putting one foot in front of the other is hard enough. "Everybody was a little bit rocky—you're the new kid at school—so it was hard to think about having to go back to college, to keep balancing school and track," Emma said. "We were all kind of like, 'This isn't exactly what we expected it to be like, but we have to go back and figure it out.' And Maddy and I were both upset with everything."

When she was with her friends, Madison found it much easier to pretend she was mostly fine. She had always been the axis around which all of them rotated, the one who directed their social calendar, made sure they ended up at the right parties. Maddy was always on her grind, when it came to both work and play. Their friend group was seven strong: Maddy was the glue. Emma was down-to-earth, genuine, an Energizer Bunny. Jackie was adventurous and spontaneous. Brooke was easygoing and carefree. Erin was work hard–play hard, like Maddy, and always up for anything. MJ was a perfectionist, also like Maddy, and her parents were the strictest.

Justine was sarcastic and funny. She and MJ split the "mom" role within the group, looking out for everyone and sometimes passing on social events because they were homebodies.

Maddy had always enjoyed going out, just like any teenager. But that holiday season, according to her friends, her partying took on an edge. Her parents had never worried about Maddy's social life, because she had never let it interfere with her schoolwork or her athletics. They knew their daughter partied, but they always said, "She plays hard, but she works hard, too."

Jim and Stacy were surprised at how quickly college had overwhelmed their daughter. "I was definitely caught off guard, because it just wasn't her," Stacy said. "I don't know, all she talked about was going to Penn, and how excited she was about it, and then here she was, and it was just not what she was expecting."

That week, they recognized that she needed to see somebody, a professional, not someone associated with the school but somebody with more experience dealing with serious mental health crises. "We saw a big change over Thanksgiving," Jim said. "I think everything got really serious. There was a shift. She had so much anxiety. It was still in the vein of 'I'm not enjoying this.' But you could also sense it was more." They found Maddy a therapist near Allendale, and she never used Penn counseling again.

Jim and Ashley drove Madison back to Penn on Sunday. The traffic on I-95 was bumper-to-bumper. Madison seemed anxious. More storm clouds had rolled in: finals. They were now only two weeks away, and she had no idea what to expect.

Active Minds

I am driving to Philadelphia to meet with the Penn students who lead the school's chapter of Active Minds, a national organization whose mission statement includes the following: "empowering students to change the perception about mental health on college campuses."

The four of us meet on the ground floor of a dormitory. We pull together two circular tables, make a figure eight, then pull up chairs at odd angles. There is much ground to cover. I want their thoughts on what life is like at Penn; whether they believe the environment at Penn is different from that at other schools; and if so, how?

I am here because Madison wanted to be, but couldn't. One night, Madison scrolled through a list of clubs at Penn. She wanted to see what else the school had to offer. She was daydreaming about the free time she would have if she stopped running, and what she might do with it. As she read through the list, she considered the description of each club and took screenshots of the ones that interested her. She clustered the images on the bottom right of her desktop: Penn Fashion Collective, Christian Students at Penn, Art Club, AsOne Global at Penn, and Active Minds.

Then she texted Ingrid:

> **Maddy:** Just went through an entire list of all the clubs at Penn. Got some solid options.

> **Ingrid:** What clubs stuck out to you?

> **Maddy:** Penn fashion collective, Christian students at penn, art club, AsOne global at penn.

Notice anything missing?

This omission is not at all surprising. A gulf seems to exist, into which thousands of college students are falling. Some are trying to get help, but the right kind of help isn't available. Some aren't even trying, because college is supposedly about being cool and having fun, and admitting feelings of anxiety, sadness, and helplessness seems like the opposite. Attending a meeting about mental health doesn't carry the same social currency as going to a frat party and posting an awesome picture on Instagram. Others know they need help, commit to finding it, and get better. But many, like Maddy, are stuck in a gray area: aware that they need something and vaguely reaching for it, but not really sure what's going on inside them.

Rates of depression and anxiety among college students are higher than ever. The specific numbers vary, depending on the study, but all show a disturbing trend. According to the American College Health Association, the suicide rate among fifteen- to twenty-four-year-olds has tripled since the 1950s. An annual survey of college freshmen found that 30 percent reported feeling overwhelmed, with that number rising to 40.5 percent among women. This is the highest percentage registered since the survey started in 1985, at which point the numbers were approximately half what they are now. One study found that an average high school student today likely deals with as much anxiety as did a psychiatric patient in the 1950s.

The numbers are eye-opening everywhere you look: 95 percent of college counseling directors said students with significant psychological problems constitute a major concern. From 1994 to 2012, the percentage of college students who sought help and were prescribed psychiatric medications rose from 9 percent (in 1994) to 17 percent (in 2000) to 20 percent (in 2003) to 25 percent (in 2006), a number that stabilized through 2012.

And here's a particularly problematic statistic: according

to the National Alliance on Mental Illness, while 7 percent of parents reported their college students experiencing mental health issues, fully 50 percent of students rated their mental health below average or poor. In other words, even those closest to college kids often have no clue how they're really feeling. The data, the papers, the surveys—they go on for hundreds of pages. And they all point to the same conclusion: a serious mental health issue exists on our college campuses.

Over the past fifteen years or so, therapists have been processing what they've been seeing and hearing. And they talk about these issues in ways that feel very human, very real. In response to the transcript of an NPR episode from 2015, "Colleges Face Soaring Mental Health Demands," a therapist with more than twenty years of experience and a student at the University of Maryland posted the following messages.

Lisa, therapist: I believe I am/we are seeing the result of the so-called "Race to Nowhere"—the achievement/ status driven culture that our kids are raised in. My clients have spent their childhoods and in particular their adolescences putting their healthy development on hold, coached and managed by parents who are so fearful and anxious about helping their children succeed that there is simply no room for their children, my clients, to begin to know themselves. When they arrive at college, the wheels come off. They are so hard on themselves, and so out of touch with what they really care about—discovering their true interests is a foreign concept. There is such a push for perfection that normal life skills (learning time management, healthy sleep habits, adult responsibilities) are not in place. Substance abuse and other methods of self-medicating are rampant. Most of my students text with their parents multiple times a day and parents regularly run interference for them. Combine this with the incessant comparisons students make of themselves to others via social media, financial burdens and dread of graduation (for after a lifetime of curated education, graduation feels like falling off a cliff) and you have a perfect storm.

DrHibiscus: I am currently a student at the University of Maryland who suffers from anxiety and depression...

I am sick and tired of hearing the facile, tired response that my generation is "soft" and has been ill equipped by coddling "helicopter parents." My parents, and those of my peers do not fit this straw man caricature and my peers are extremely hard-working, intelligent, and ambitious. I went to weekly group therapy provided by my school's Counseling Center last year. What I learned about myself and about my peers was that our main source of stress was that we were simply not allowed to be human...My generation is not suffering because we didn't learn how to lose a game of flag football. We're suffering because everything we do is filtered through a lens of consumerism. We see ourselves as "products" to be "branded" and "marketed" in all venues of our lives: social, romantic, and professional. This has been a mindset inculcated into us from an early age.

EVERYTHING we do is seen as instrumental towards marketing ourselves for the college admission boards, or for the job market, or to help us rush a fraternity or sorority, or to help us win friends, or to help us be a more attractive potential partner. You see the capitalist worldview has infiltrated our psychology, and our sense of self-worth. And it is toxic. It results in fear of being ourselves and following what we really want to do. It results in micro-managing every aspect of our lives to best effect so that it looks good for Facebook or LinkedIn or Tinder. It results in constant comparisons with our peers (which causes depression) and catastrophizing of any potential dent to our marketability (which results in anxiety). Essentially, it results in a dehumanized mindset.

Of course depression and anxiety are rampant.

In 2014, Penn commissioned a task force to assess the climate on campus and how this climate might affect students.

The eight-page report used the term "destructive perfection-ism" and observed that "the drive for academic excellence along with the perception that in order to be successful one needs to hold leadership roles in multiple realms contributes to the amount of stress and distress experienced by Penn students."

This last quote is essentially a description of the "Penn Face," which is the phrase used to describe the culture of appearing effortlessly perfect. It's a concept that the three leaders of Active Minds very much want to talk about. All experienced it, and continue experiencing it, and all believe that variations of the concept likely exist on campuses across the country. Each of the three students at the table—Kathryn DeWitt, Peter Moon, Devanshi Mehta—reached out to Active Minds because they were struggling to varying degrees with their emotional and mental well-being. And the climate at Penn contributed to that struggle.

> **Devanshi:** I think Penn students coined the phrase "Penn Face" to represent how everyone gives off a certain image of being okay, and having every-thing together, and almost, like, say, even though I'm stressed, I still have time to have a perfect social life, perfect grades, to join all these clubs, and I'm super successful. But in reality people are stressed, and do feel alone, and it's important to address those things.

Peter: Picture a duck, and below the surface they are scrambling for their lives, but above the water everything appears peaceful—not a care in the world. That's Penn Face.

Kathryn: I think Penn Face also comes from the expectations we have for ourselves, and that people around us have for us at an Ivy League university— you're supposed to be having the best four years of your life. We get this messaging everywhere. And having a hard time is not part of that messaging, which perpetuates the belief that "I'm not okay" must mean that something is wrong with you instead of something a lot of people might feel.

Devanshi: Ivy League schools compile all the top students in one place and then all of a sudden you look left and right and you're like, "Everyone is my clone." I literally got here and I was like, "I'm not unique, I am not special, I am just like everyone else." The culture here, the first week of school, the library is packed, everyone is studying. That was my identity in high school—she's a hard worker. And I came here and it's like, "Who am I?" And it manifested itself in anxiety and sadness. I didn't feel comfortable with who I was anymore.

(Here, Devanshi is cutting to the core of something specific. On one hand, the job of parents is to make their child
feel special and unique, as if they can do anything they put
their mind to. After all, if our parents don't believe in us, who
will? But instilling those beliefs in a child is healthy only if
balanced with a reality check about what the world is like,
about how hard and difficult it can be, and about how few
people will likely ascribe those same qualities of uniqueness
and wonder to you. Somewhere along the way, we've started
to believe that delivering this second message is cruel. But it's
not. Cruelty is offering either message — without the other.)

Kathryn: It's like, if you have a sprained ankle, you
can say that you have one and people say, "Yeah,
that makes sense why you're in pain right now."
But if you say you're depressed, nobody really wants
to talk about that, or believe it's a real thing. Also,
the competition here is awful.

Peter: And it's made harder because the person you
perceive yourself as competing with is trying so
hard to be modest about it, like it's no big deal.

Devanshi: Just so nonchalant about it.

Devanshi: And it's a very preprofessional school.
You're put into this environment where people
don't just have their major figured out, but supposedly

have their life figured out—even the next ten years planned out. So if you don't, it's like, "Well, what am I even doing?"

As a freshman in 2014, Kathryn actually planned her suicide. She had written dozens of goodbye letters to friends and family; she'd even picked the location. "It's never just one thing that leads someone to that place," she said. "It's multiple factors. It felt like everyone else had their lives together and no one else was feeling so alone, struggling so much, and having all these identity questions. I didn't see a way out. I didn't see a way to live up to my expectations, my parents' expectations, my friends' expectations."

But then in the days before she could carry out her plan, the resident advisor in her dorm—the same one where Madison lived, in fact—staged an intervention. The woman did so because everyone in the dorm was discussing warning signs of depression. Essentially, they were on high alert. Kathryn took a leave of absence and returned to Penn a year later. In the time since, she's read everything she can about mental health, including the current state of college counseling—at Penn and elsewhere.

In the past three years, Penn has improved its counseling system. The upgrade was in response to the fact that six students, including Madison, died by suicide during a thirteen-month period, from 2013 to 2014. The tragedies led to a task force, which led to the hiring of additional counselors and the counseling center moving to a bigger space. The improvements allowed the school to cut its wait time for an initial appointment from 13.2 days (the average from 2012 to 2013) to just two to three. Yet even as Penn has attempted to improve its counseling services, as well as to acknowledge its on-campus culture, suicides have continued: six additional students have taken their lives since 2014, approximately twice the national average.

This problem, this crush of struggling students, is not unique to Penn. Colleges across the country are dealing with an overload of cases. The counseling centers of many universities are staffed and funded at essentially the same level they were twenty years ago, before the rise in the number of students with mental health issues. For a long time, college counseling centers were adequate. Students who needed help with issues big or small could easily schedule an appointment. Over the past ten years, though, on many college campuses these spaces have morphed into the equivalent of an overtrafficked emergency room. According to the American Psychological Association, 76.6 percent of counseling center directors said they are having to reduce the number of visits with noncrisis patients in order to cope with the growing number of cases. There's a name for that practice: it's called triage.

Exactly when do our young people have time to develop their own sense of self? When are they able to be alone, to understand how they think, what they really want—without the pretense of how it might look on a college application?

And we're not just talking high school students; this practice of hovering often begins before they've learned how to write. Kids used to grow up in the neighborhood—on the block or in the parks, playing games with other kids. These games had rules, but the kids themselves determined them, flexing their imaginations. Social scientists call these activities—capture the flag, bike races, pickup baseball games—"free play," and it's been steadily decreasing since the 1950s. Scientists have also noted a correlation between the decreasing amount of childhood free play—any play not directed by adults—and the increasing rates of anxiety and depression among kids. As free play decreases, anxiety increases. Correlation does not equal causation, but considering that free play helps kids develop their sense of self, their problem-solving abilities, their ability to self-soothe, and their ability to play well with others, it's not a stretch to see why scientists believe the decrease in free play is possibly affecting their mental health.

In the article "The Decline of Play and the Rise of Pathology," which appeared in the *American Journal of Play,* author Peter Gray cites the work of psychologist Jean Twenge, who discusses how too many kids are chasing goals over which they have minimal control. Gray writes:

> Developing competence at an activity that one enjoys, making friends, finding meaning in life, and pursuing a heartfelt religious path are examples of intrinsic goals. Getting high grades in school, making lots of money, achieving high status, and looking good to others are examples of extrinsic goals. Twenge argues convincingly that there has been a continual shift away from intrinsic toward extrinsic values in the culture at large and among young people in particular, promoted in part by the mass marketing of consumer goods through television and other media. She refers also to evidence that the pursuit of extrinsic goals at the expense of intrinsic goals correlates with anxiety and depression. It seems reasonable that this would be true.

Gray later writes: "Humans are extraordinarily adaptive to changes in their living conditions, but not infinitely so." Now add in social media. Is there anything you have less control over than how many likes you receive on a photo? As scholar William Deresiewicz has written, we have created a generation of world-class hoop jumpers, of "excellent sheep," of young people who know what they're supposed to say, but not necessarily why they're saying it. We're teaching young people *what* to think, but not *how* to think. Deresiewicz writes:

> Introspection means talking to yourself, and one of the best ways of talking to yourself is by talking to another person. One other person you can trust, one other person to whom you can unfold your soul. One other person you feel safe enough with to allow you to acknowledge things—to acknowledge things to yourself—that you otherwise can't. Doubts you aren't supposed to have, questions you aren't supposed to ask. Feelings or opinions that would get you laughed at by the group or reprimanded by the authorities.
>
> This is what we call thinking out loud, discovering what you believe in the course of articulating it. But it takes just as much time and just as much patience as solitude in the strict sense. And our new electronic world has disrupted it just as violently. Instead of having one or two true friends that we can sit and talk to for three hours at a time, we have 968 "friends" that we never actually talk to; instead we just bounce one-line messages off them a hundred times a day. This is not friendship, this is distraction.

Kathryn, the Penn student who works with Active Minds, is sitting across from me. She has brought printouts, all kinds of information she wants to share, numbers and studies and articles. She has thought of all the angles affecting this issue, the collision of events that has brought us here. Sometimes it seems as if an easy answer is just around the corner, but then when you get there, a switchback appears.

She knows that, back when she was a freshman, having someone to whom she could unfold her soul would have made life easier. But who finds that person within months of arriving in a new city, at a new school? Who can find a soul mate when her own soul is still such a work in progress?

"Nobody here knows you from before, knows who you are and how you act," Kathryn said. "So nobody really knows if you're different, or if there's something really wrong, because the truth is, they don't know you at all."

At least now, Kathryn has the friends sitting around this table. And while that does not make everything better, it does make one thing better. She knows for certain she is not the only one feeling this way.

CHAPTER 5

Just Sleep

The night of December 12, Madison texted her dad *I need to come home*. Immediately he wrote her back, told her to book the first train out of Philadelphia the following morning. He would pick her up at the Newark station. Track practice, studying for finals, those things were secondary; most important was that they see her, talk, put some sort of plan in motion to fix whatever was happening. Later they could figure out the logistics of what she might miss.

Everything had escalated so quickly in her mind. How had that happened? She had been fending off the worst thoughts for weeks, the ones she knew she shouldn't be having. She'd been focusing instead on ways to calm herself, to make things better. But the worst thoughts were persistent, bold, incessantly tugging at her consciousness. She really didn't want to let them in. But at some point she did, convincing herself that she could open the door just a sliver, just to take a break from the constant knocking. Maybe the thoughts would come in and sit still. In a backward way, the worst thoughts actually calmed her. They were reassuring, like knowing that there was a secret escape route in case the room caught fire. Of course, there was a chance that these thoughts might destroy everything, actually set the room on fire. Was that what was happening? Or did the fire already exist?

Over the past few weeks—each time practice, or studying for final exams, or looking at someone else's beautiful and carefree Instagram feed, like those of the Penn seniors whose friendships seemed everlasting, hadn't gone well—those worst thoughts would begin to boil. They did not obey. They did not just simmer in the background. And they were offering something clear-cut: a way out.

Suicide. That word felt heavy and sharp, impossible for Madison to even think about, let alone say out loud. Everything else in her mind felt abstract, so abstract that Maddy felt immobilized by the lack of clarity. Where had all this darkness come from? Her mind had always been a wilderness, but a mostly well-lit one, so she could see her footing. But now shadows had settled over parts, blackness rolling into all the crevices. Peeking around corners felt dangerous.

The scariest part was that out of this foggy world would occasionally come one slice of frightening clarity. Thoughts, so purposeful and disciplined, would burst through like a train cutting through a snowstorm, an iron fist on a collision course with its destination. Maddy had, in fact, thought of the power of such a train—a real one. And thought also of how defenseless she would be standing in its path. What would that feel like? Would it be exhilarating? In a single moment, a cold, inhuman force could turn fear into fearlessness. At least, maybe that's how others would see it, would see her, instead of the soul-crushing panic she actually felt.

According to one close friend, she was thinking of this train. She thought of walking onto the tracks, just a mile or two down the road. She couldn't go to the 30th Street Station, with its marble floors and vaulted ceilings, because trains were either idle there or pulling into or out of the building, so slow as to be harmless. She thought instead about the stretch of track that ran parallel to the Schuylkill, the river that separated University City from Center City. In Dutch, Schuylkill literally means "hidden river," so the easy way to tell locals from outsiders is whether they add the word "river" after Schuylkill: the hidden river river. Maddy had learned this fact upon first moving to Philly. The tracks were near Penn, down an embankment, and trains had usually picked up steam by the time they passed through.

She thought of leaving her dorm room, of those final minutes, of the relief gained by making such a clear and decisive choice. God—what was she even talking about? Who owned this new voice inside her?

This couldn't happen. She desperately needed her mom and dad.

That morning, December 13, as she rode Amtrak home, she sent an e-mail to her assistant coach, Robin Martin, explaining why she would miss practice that afternoon:

From: Madison Holleran
To: Robin Martin

Hi coach Martin! I have some bad news. I woke up this morning feeling very very sick and threw up a lot. I don't know what exactly is wrong but my parents thought it'd be best for me to come home for the weekend and rest for finals. I'm taking the train home soon so I obviously won't be at practice today. I don't know how this happened :(hope practice goes well and I'll see you soon!

From: Robin Martin
To: Madison Holleran

No worries. Get better!

Before sending the e-mail to Martin, Maddy texted a number of her friends, letting them know that whatever plans she had made with them for the rest of that week, she couldn't keep. Each text was almost identical to the others and paralleled the story she'd told Martin.

> **Maddy:** Hi friend!! I hope you aced your math final!! Just wanted to let you know I'm going home for the weekend. Woke up feeling so sick And threw up a lot and my parents thought it would be best to come home and rest so I'm getting on a train now

Ingrid: Oh my god I'm so sorry!! Are you feeling any better? I wish I could do something to help!!

Of course, Ingrid could not help. Perhaps she could have, perhaps she would have said and done just the right thing—if she'd known the real problem. But she thought Maddy needed things you could buy at the store, deflated ginger ale and Tylenol, and maybe a fun party to take her mind off track practices. But what was the fix if you needed to take your mind off...your mind?

Jim met Maddy at the Newark station. She climbed into the front seat of the Ford. He looked at his daughter, looked quickly away. What had happened? She had been home for

Thanksgiving not three weeks before. Things hadn't been great, but they weren't like this. He put the car into gear, turned the wheel, looked back at her.

"Madison," he said. "I think you look depressed."

He didn't know how else to describe her. He was sure, in that moment, that the word he had used was not hyperbole, but precise, necessary. She leaned back in the seat. Her head touched the headrest. She was wearing a sweatshirt, her hair pulled back. All the color that was once in her cheeks had migrated to the rims of her eyes. When she spoke, her voice, usually high, was low, as if forming words took energy she didn't have.

"Dad," she whispered, "all I want to do is go to sleep."

"Let's get you home," he said.

Madison walked through the front door and immediately went upstairs to lie down. Jim wasn't sure what to expect from her over the next few days. Rather, he didn't have expectations. He was just relieved she was beneath their roof. He and Stacy discussed what was happening, how different their daughter seemed, how concerned they were. "We need to start getting her consistent professional help—as quickly as we can," they agreed. They called the therapist they had connected with over Thanksgiving break, scheduled an appointment for that weekend. Maddy surprised them when she came downstairs just an hour later. She was dressed in workout clothes, her sneakers on.

"I want to go join a gym," she said. She was going to be

home that weekend, also over winter break after finals, and she needed a place to stay in shape for the next month, she explained. Just a few hours earlier, opening the car door seemed to have exhausted her, but now she was determined to burn energy as if she possessed an endless supply.

This had become the cycle, the endless battle: like carrying a weight on her shoulders, then finally dropping to her knees because it was too much, then telling herself not to be weak, to get up as she always had, to find a way to keep moving forward. Then she would stand, tell herself she could handle this, and start walking again. Until, of course, she would again collapse beneath the weight.

This sequence was not unlike high-intensity intervals on the track. And, just like those, each repetition took more effort than the previous one. That was actually the point of interval training: raising your heart rate to 180, then dropping it to resting, then raising it again—this drained energy much faster than maintaining a steady pace. How many more intervals could she run? She wasn't sure, but she had to keep getting up, because perhaps the next one would be the last, perhaps the weight would disappear as quickly as it had appeared.

Jim drove Maddy to Retro Fitness, a few miles away on Route 17, and they signed her up for a monthlong membership. Sometimes she ran on the treadmill, other times she sat on the bike for dozens of miles, sweat dripping across the display, her head down and legs churning through hills. She needed the endorphins. The rush of them made her feel like herself, even if it was fleeting, even if she could often feel the sensation leaking from her body before she pulled on her sweats and opened the door to leave the gym. The alternative was lying in her bed, staring at the ceiling, and just hoping and praying that something would change. But that wasn't her—that had never been her. She wanted to keep doing the things that had once made her feel good. And so instead of sleeping in her childhood bed, turning from side to side, letting the exhaustion wash over her, drown her, she decided to get up and put on her sneakers. She would keep making that choice. Maybe she could churn out the darkness, force it to seep out of her, like sweat, if she just ran fast enough, long enough.

That first evening, she spent a couple hours at the gym. While there, she got a text from her high school friend Erin: "Going over to your house!" Erin did not know that Maddy was home from school, but she had just finished finals and was home for winter break. She was close to Ashley Holleran, who was back from Alabama, as well as the rest of the Holleran family. When she texted, Erin thought Maddy was still at Penn, so she was surprised when she got a message back that said, "I'm at the gym, be back soon."

Erin and another of Ashley's friends, Brandon, were at the Hollerans' when Maddy walked through the door. Erin was expecting to see the person she remembered from high school, the Maddy who was laughing and happy, the Maddy who would bolt up the stairs to shower, then come back down ready to hear all about what had happened during first semester. But that person did not walk through the door. Erin couldn't quite figure out what was happening. Maddy seemed evasive, avoiding eye contact as if she had something to hide. She quickly excused herself.

Erin had just spent seven days in the library, studying for finals, so she reminded herself how anxious and tired she had felt during that time. That's all this was. Maddy was still in the middle of it all, cramming for her first-ever Ivy League exams. And anyway, it was late at night. The whole interaction was understandable, explainable even. It was dark out, and Erin was seeing Maddy in the artificial light of the room, so maybe it was a kind of optical illusion. Maybe she wasn't quite as pale and empty as she looked.

Over the next few days, Jim and Stacy tried to understand exactly what was going on, but Madison seemed incapable of articulating what she was feeling. She kept falling back on the stress of finals, and how she felt she was failing multiple courses. And when she wasn't talking about that anxiety, she simply kept saying, "Something is wrong, something is really wrong."

They soon believed that the solution to their daughter's struggle was beyond their purview, which as parents they found hard to accept. They felt that only a highly trained professional could help Maddy. "She had a really hard time

132 • WHAT MADE MADDY RUN

talking about what was going on," Jim said. "I think she was really confused. Honestly, I wasn't sure what was going on exactly. I just knew that I couldn't help her. I felt that she needed a psychologist, or somebody that was really well trained and qualified. And we had insurance through my work, so we knew she was covered."

Madison wanted the help. Mostly. Her worst thoughts were encouraging her to reject help, to keep the feelings to herself. The creature seemed to want to convince her that she needed to find a solution on her own, that she was becoming burdensome to those around her, to her family.

Mackenzie was a junior at Highlands; Brendan was a freshman. Just as, one year earlier, Madison could not comprehend why Ashley was unhappy at Penn State, Mackenzie could not fathom why Maddy was so miserable at Penn. Wasn't college all Madison had talked about? When they were growing up, every time she yelled at Mack for borrowing one of her tops or a pair of her jeans, Maddy would talk about how she would soon be out of the house, off to somewhere much more exciting and interesting, where she wouldn't have to deal with such an annoying little sister.

As much as it seemed from the outside that they were always fighting, that was only because they were so much alike. Beneath the façade of feuding sisters, they had laid the groundwork for a great friendship. Before Maddy left for Penn, she wrote Mackenzie a letter:

Mackenzie

I am so thankful to call you my sister. You are gorgeous (yes I admit it), talented, mature (for the most part), responsible, modest, and so fun to be around. I know these aren't things you hear from me often but they are the honest truth. And I know I yell at you a lot but most of the time I don't mean to, it's just what I'm used to ... so I'm sorry for that. Can't believe you're 16 years old and I also cannot believe we won't be living together anymore in just over a month. The thought of not being under the same roof as each other is actually scary to me. Not going to lie, I'm already a tad bit nervous. You better be prepared to visit me frequently because as much as I hate to admit it, I will miss you a lot. I'm proud of the person you have become and how much you've matured over the years. The amount that you've changed just since you started out at Highlands is insane ... Remember to always keep your head up no matter how many times people try to put you down. "You're braver than you believe, stronger than you seem, and smarter than you think." There's a lot I will miss about you when I go off to college. I will miss singing (belting out) country songs together. I will miss watching the Voice together and having you yell at me every time I speak. I will miss making fun of Jimbo together. I will miss our trips to Starbucks every Monday and Friday before school. I will miss trying to break into Ashley's closet to steal her clothes. I will miss your annoying and infectious laugh. But I can't wait to come back home and hear about all of the latest Highlands gossip. Maybe when I come home you will actually have a BOYFRIEND. That'd be cray now wouldn't it ;). I know you are only halfway done with high school but I'm telling you, embrace every second of it because it's over in the blink of an eye. Stay focused throughout Junior year in regards to schoolwork, tennis and track but live it up as well. Don't party as hard as I did (do?) but it's ok to go a lil crazy at times. Even though I'll be in Philly and away at college, I'll always be here for you. LOVE YOU YA CRAZY SKANK RASCAL HOE MUNCHKIN.

Love, ur fav, obviously...Madison.

A week before unexpectedly taking the train home, Maddy had texted with her younger sister, seemingly trying to connect, to share her pain. But Mackenzie couldn't quite grasp how college—that place of adulthood, freedom, dreams—could be making her sister unhappy. Like many such connection failures, this was actually a failure of imagination.

Mackenzie and others pictured college in one way; Madison experienced it in another.

Mack: How is it

          Maddy: How is what

Mack: Penn

          Maddy: It sucks Mackenzie

          Maddy: It sucks so much

Mack: What are you doing rn

          Maddy: Going to dinner

Mack: With who

          Maddy: My friend Eleanor. I can't do this anymore

          Maddy: I hate this place

Mack: Why r u so miserable

          Maddy: It's everything especially track

          Maddy: I hate it so much

Mack: Do u have fun at party's

Maddy: Not really

Mack: Do u get with people

Maddy: Not rlly

Madison had to return to Philly for a few days to finish finals and to complete first semester. Jim and Stacy reassured her that her time in Philly was temporary, and that she would be back home the following week, with an entire month to figure out what was happening. All she needed to do was manage for a few days, and then she could come right back to Allendale. "In high school, everything that could go right for Madison, did," says Mackenzie. "High school wasn't a struggle for her, so it was hard to understand how college had so quickly gone bad. With track, she got to be the best because of how hard she worked. She got a 4.0 in school because she studied so much. And she was even partying less in college. I wanted to visit her, and she said that she only goes out one night a week in college. I was surprised. She started going out less, started doing everything less."

All Alone

The first night I started writing this book, I spent ten hours in front of Madison's computer. I had driven the hour from Brooklyn to Allendale that afternoon, to the Hollerans' home, where Ashley was waiting for me, MacBook in hand. Madison's computer was Brendan's now, but her account had been preserved and was just a few keystrokes away. Thankfully, Brendan was willing to part with the device for the weekend.

On the TV that night was *Thursday Night Football:* Denver vs. Kansas City. I remember glancing at the New York City skyline and feeling a burst of gratitude, a frequent emotion of mine, that I lived in such a dynamic place. At another point, I remember reaching over to rest my hand on the leg of my girlfriend. Other than these two brief moments, I lived inside a screen. Time passed imperceptibly, the way it does when you zone out while driving, the miles rolling along, and then the gas light dings and you can't remember having covered a long stretch of road.

On Madison's computer I looked through photographs. I accessed (with the help of her family) her Gmail and University of Pennsylvania accounts, scrolling back through years of messages. As I carefully looked through everything, the blue iMessage icon containing all Madison's text messages loomed on the dashboard. The icon seemed to radiate energy. I was saving it for last. Or maybe I was avoiding it—scared of what clues it might or might not contain.

I was reconstructing Madison, which meant simultaneously deconstructing myself. To be fully present in Maddy's online world, I had to absent myself from my own. I was building Maddy more clearly—her thoughts, her important moments—from the data on a screen, drawing whole ideas and even conclusions from fragments of her thinking, from the slivers of herself that she dared expose to the world. Using the deluge of information held in that computer, I was building a portrait to make Maddy come alive. In attempting this, I became for varying lengths of time someone who wasn't.

We're all doing exactly this, all the time now. Even before I began learning about Madison, I had started the process of erasing myself from the present world in favor of social media—carving out chunks of myself, stretching them into an online skeleton: two people from one, like some kind of medical miracle. I had been doing this for a long time, of my own volition. In the past few years, I've spent almost as much time constructing and maintaining my online self as I have my real, human self. I've certainly spent more time on Instagram exercising my image than I have in the gym exercising my body.

These two presentations are not the same person; in fact, they are often two very different people. The online version is static, and therefore easily paused on perfection, because the conditions in that space allow it. The parameters of the actual world are expansive, and people can view you from any angle (literally and metaphorically), while online you need only fit yourself into a fixed box whose conditions you control and manipulate. The offline version of me is obviously deeply flawed, though it's easy to start believing otherwise, because I spend so much time immersed in my online self. Online, I can create someone who is not impatient, does not misspeak, is not self-centered, is always standing in the best lighting, and on and on. The highlights of my life are posted in that space, and everyone reacts in predictable ways — that is, the ways I want them to. And sometimes it feels much easier to live in that reality than in the one where I am always flawed and challenged, and occasionally sad.

So what do these two versions of me have in common? Honestly, not much at all. For example, imagine that over the course of a year I posted images of sentences from this book online, and after seeing several hundred of them, you started to believe that you knew what the book was about, its energy and message. Imagine that you then actually got hold of the book and read it cover to cover. Perhaps I had carefully selected passages that reflected the whole—that's possible. More likely, though, I had selected passages that made the book seem interesting, that put forth the story line or narrative I liked best. The book could seem like a romance but actually be horror, or it could seem like suspense but actually be comedy, or it could seem well written but actually be a mess. You've no clue.

I imagine this is true for almost everyone's social persona, Madison included. One of the trickiest parts of social media is recognizing that everyone is doing the same thing you're doing: presenting their best self. Everyone is now a brand, and all of digital life is a fashion magazine. While it's easy to understand intrinsically that your presence on social media is only one small sliver of your full story, it's more difficult to apply that logic to everyone else. Because you actually lived the full night, not just the two-second snapshot of everyone laughing, arms around shoulders. All you see of other people's nights is an endless string of laughing snapshots, which your brain easily extrapolates to fantastic evenings filled with warmth and love, with good wine and delicious food. Comparing your everyday existence to someone else's highlight reel is dangerous for both of you.

At the same time, existing online often feels less risky, less challenging, than existing in the real world, where things often become messy. Online, you can just plug in and edit everything. Plus, there is no body language that you're forced to interpret. When you try to build a relationship in person, or meet a group of friends, you face the possibility of awkward pauses, confusing body language, and the disappointment of not saying precisely what you mean. In person, time moves steadily past and you either keep the rhythm of the interaction or you don't. Online, there is only the artificial rhythm you create, the beat slowed down or sped up depending on what you choose. But that's not quite dancing. Dancing is giving your body over to a larger energy. Dancing is finding the rhythm and beauty in whatever song is playing.

It's easier to feel connected online than to truly connect in real life. So plugging in becomes addicting. We'd rather sign on and feel some superficial sense of connection than work and possibly fail at true connection offline. Being in the real world can be uncomfortable, especially after you spend so much time online.

"Split Image," my espnW story about Madison's life and her death, went online while I was sitting alone in a small room with the door closed. I was perched on a chair, bright lights overhead, staring into a camera, preparing to tape *Around the*

Horn. Yet all I could think about was the story, which for nearly a year existed only in my head or on my computer screen, but now also existed on other people's screens, in other people's heads. Would anyone feel what I felt? What would they think? How would the story make them feel?

I hit Send on a tweet I'd spent an hour writing, the tweet like a carrier pigeon swooping across the Internet with the story's link. And between the taping of each block of *Around the Horn,* I refreshed Twitter. Had anyone finished the piece yet? Did they care enough to respond? As I walked out of the ESPN Times Square building after filming, I kept refreshing, and the following sentence is not much of an exaggeration: I did not stop refreshing Twitter for five months. At night, for hours, I would rotate loading Twitter, then Instagram, Gmail, and iMessage. I stopped reading books because I couldn't concentrate; I would launch my phone after reading each page. I rarely called people on the phone, but I sent thousands of texts, many with emojis. The point is, even before I lost myself trying to reconstruct Maddy, I had already lost myself to some hollow online version of me. The volume of the response to "Split Image," as well as the intensity of the messages, felt like a kind of drug. For weeks, every time I refreshed my e-mail or Twitter, I got a hit of dopamine. And so in the months afterward, I continued to feverishly refresh those accounts, hoping for more digital feedback and interaction.

In her book *Mind Change,* Susan Greenfield asks this relevant question: *"What if a cyber airbrushed persona started to elbow out the real you?"* It's easy to imagine your social persona as the most polished version of yourself. In the 1800s, this would be the "you" that showed up at the ball, or the dance, or Christmas Day service: best clothes, best face, ready to charm. And of course there's nothing radical about presenting edited versions of ourselves, which we've always done. We once sent letters by horseback that contained only the words and ideas we wanted relayed. We once commissioned artists to paint our likeness, and these paintings almost certainly incorporated the equivalent of filters, specific instructions to paint the subject in the best possible light, from the best angle—soften the features, please. Self-editing began at the beginning. The only difference now is the volume of one another's edited lives that we consume.

In December 2016, *The New Yorker* posted an article by Jia Tolentino, "The Worst Year Ever, Until Next Year." In it, Tolentino addresses the potential, yet still unknowable, problems created by digital consumption. "There is no limit to the amount of misfortune a person can take in via the Internet," she writes. "And there's no easy way to properly calibrate it—no guidebook for how to expand your heart to accommodate these simultaneous scales of human experience; no way to train your heart to separate the banal from the profound. Our ability to change things is not increasing at the same rate as our ability to know about them. No, 2016 is not the worst year ever, but it's the year I started feeling like the Internet would only ever induce the sense of power-lessness that comes when the sphere of what a person can influence remains static, while the sphere of what can influence us seems to expand without limit, allowing no respite at all."

Before social media, we mostly interacted with one an-other in the bright light of day, where we all have so much less control over how we might look or seem. Now we spend hours a day consuming one another online. Moreover, digital natives have known only this reality. They have grown up on Instagram and Snapchat, absorbing hundreds of images a day. And most of these perfect pictures, loaded into boxes, reflect little of each person's reality. We're consuming an increas-ingly filtered world yet walking through our own realities unfiltered.

Maybe this matters less when life is good. Maybe when we're in a good space, when we're "happy," it's nice to launch social media and see how well everyone else is doing. The whole experience might feel like momentum, all this beauty and goodness gracefully stacking higher and higher. And when you're in this place, you're often rational, too, because your mind isn't in fight-or-flight mode. Your pulse is low. Your thinking is clear. You're able to recognize how edited so much of it is. *But that's okay,* you tell yourself, because life is so good, and beautiful pictures and projected happiness are lovely.

But how often are we in that sane and safe place? And what about the rest of the time, when life is cloudy and gray, and getting out of your head is a struggle? Then what impact does the perfectly manicured landscape of social media have on our brains? A study of more than seven hundred college students by researchers at the University of Missouri found that Facebook could spark feelings of envy, which can lead to symptoms of depression. When you're anxious and low, and out of habit (and addiction) you launch social media, it is unlikely that images of others will help you feel connected. Rather, they almost certainly further pry apart the space between you and everyone else, because you are not happy and everyone else seems to be.

Social media has psychological side effects. Paradoxically, hyperconnectivity may create feelings of disconnection — not only between us and others, but within ourselves. In *Mind Change,* clinical psychologist Larry Rosen points out that a "dangerous gap could grow between this idealized 'front stage' you and the real 'backstage' you, leading to a feeling of disconnection and isolation." Social media doesn't represent the first chance we've had to "distort" our identity, but it is the first that allows us to do so in such volume, and with such accessibility. Many celebrities have long felt the extreme disconnect between the public and private versions of themselves. Now the lived experience of a fractured persona, and the emotional impact of it, is being felt to varying degrees by millions of us.

This potential "division" within ourselves is compounded by a decrease in our attention spans and depth of thinking. Throughout human history, we have soothed ourselves by creating, by mining our brains and hearts, turning pain into thoughts, thoughts into art. Now we are tethered to a steady hum of the superficial, and it is becoming increasingly difficult to disconnect, to turn inward, away from that buzz. Even our sense of time has shape-shifted, because everything can be accessed instantaneously. It's not hard to see, when viewed through this lens, that carefully considered responses are being replaced by knee-jerk reactions.

Another addition to this technological whirlwind: texting and emojis. Social media and texting have something specific in common: they both allow you to easily create a version of yourself that is more palatable—to others and to yourself. Texting gives the user ultimate control. A face-to-face conversation, or even a telephone call, might reveal more than someone intends or desires. Like water, verbal communication is hard to contain, easily spilling over. On text, users answer only what they want to answer and can easily end the conversation abruptly if they don't like where it's going. Or for any reason at all. In her book *Alone Together,* Sherry Turkle writes that young people "prefer to deal with strong feelings from the safe haven of the Net. It gives them an alternative to processing emotions in real time."

Young adults now predominantly communicate through text, or on Instagram and Snapchat. All of us, adults included, call people on the phone less frequently. Text is absolutely an efficient mode of staying in touch, because we can engage with numerous people while working—a steady stream of contact. And again, this may be fine when you're feeling healthy and happy. But when you're not, studies show that relying on these modes of digital communication does little to curb feelings of isolation and sadness.

Efficient communication does not mean effective communication. Our perception of efficacy is dependent on our desired outcome. We communicate for many different reasons: sometimes merely to make plans, sometimes out of boredom or duty, and other times because we are struggling and need compassion and empathy. Most worrisome are the ways social media complicates or reduces our ability to reach one another when we're in distress.

Consider this passage from *Mind Change:* "Teenagers who spoke with their parents over the phone or in person released similar amounts of oxytocin [an indication of bonding and well-being] and showed similar low levels of cortisol [a marker of stress], indicative of a reduction in stress. In comparison, those who instant-messaged their parents released no oxytocin and had salivary cortisol levels as high as those who did not interact with their parents at all. Thus while the younger generation may favor non-oral modes of communication, when it comes to providing emotional support, messaging appears comparable to not speaking with anyone at all."

Finally, after searching every crevice of Madison's computer, I slowly moved the mouse to the dashboard and hovered over the blue iMessage icon. If someone accessed my iMessage file, they would find a blow-by-blow account of my days, as there are numerous people with whom I keep in pretty much constant contact. I'm also relatively forthcoming—at least with my close friends—about how I'm feeling. So while certain details are of course omitted (everyone has their secrets), the texts would provide a transparent view of my thinking, my mental state. I wondered whether Madison's would provide the same.

I launched the application. Months and months of messages popped onto the screen. Suddenly I felt overwhelmed, as if I were staring into a cluttered garage with no idea where to find what I was looking for. Perhaps Maddy sent something meaningful a month ago to a friend she never texted again, an exchange buried beneath more recent interactions. I pictured a block of blue text, the words capturing everything going through Madison's mind. Meticulous work would reveal this long-buried clue.

I started reading the conversations with her closest friends, those whose names I knew, because their communication happened to be more recent. Only a few minutes passed before I realized that I would not find anything insightful within Madison's iMessage account. In fact, the most important realization I would arrive at was how superficial the medium could be. She sent thousands of messages, perhaps ten thousand words—and yet little was actually said.

We have this idea that someone's phone will reveal their life, that if you found an iPhone on the street you'd have access to photos, e-mail, notes, texts, videos, apps. Each of these would project an angle of light that would gradually illuminate a whole person. But the truth is nothing like that. The truth is that a phone will help you build something like a hologram, and if you tried to touch it, your hand would breeze right through the image.

Still, I looked through every last one of Madison's messages. After about an hour of clicking on names, reading, then clicking out, I launched an exchange with another friend, and my hands froze over the keyboard. My heart banged inside my chest. There, in the text box, were five words Maddy had typed but never sent—*hey, what are you doing*—followed by a blinking cursor. It was the cursor that caused my heart to race. The thin line seemed to be alive, waiting for Madison's next move, like a blinking red traffic light at which she was idling, looking both ways, considering where to go next.

I thought, *Wow, this is like having Madison, right here in front of me.*

But is it really?

CHAPTER 6

Size Nothing

This isn't a goodbye letter/Even if Emma wanted to say bye I wouldn't let her/Because she is a friend forever, that I can bet her/I could say that ever since the day I met her/ She doesn't only remember me as the bed wetter./

Realistically, at this point in my life, there aren't a whole lot of people who I consider lifelong friends, who I want to remain close with until the day I die, who I can trust with all my heart; but you are one of the few. Ever since the second grade I have considered you one of my best friends, and year after year our friendship gradually strengthened. I can include several other people in that last sentence, but there is a distinct difference between you and the rest. You and I have been through EVERYTHING together. Even though we've only had one class together in ALL of high school, we've still become closer than I could have imagined. We've relied on each other, cried with each other, yelled at each other (blame it on the alc...), helped each other, and grown into the people we are today because we've had each other along the way. Whether it's on the soccer field, on the track, or in life outside of sports, I can always count on you. My favorite part about our friendship is that I've seen you change more than almost any other person since the day I met you, yet you've always remained the same Emma. You've always stayed true to yourself and lived by your own morals, not anyone else's. But even though I know you and your morals, LET LOOSE AND GO CRAY IN COLLEGE!! Whose a single lady? Eeemmmmmmmmaaaaaaa.

Emma,

this may be one of the hardest letters I have ever written to someone. I want to start off by saying thank you. Thank you for being there for me through it all and never letting me down. Thank you for being an absolutely amazing friend. When I think of the qualities a good friend should have, I realized that you possess all of them. Loyal, trustworthy, caring, fun-loving, easy to talk to. If I ever had a problem or needed someone to talk to I knew I could come to you about anything. And when I think of all the most memorable times these four years have brought, you were right there with me. From being on the greatest team in the world, NHGS, to surprising ourselves and becoming All-Americans in track, we shared those unforgettable moments. We even shared some of our worst moments, and when the going got rough, not once did we give up on each other. Even though I don't recall the majority of the night, and I'm sure you don't either, if I remember just one thing from Claire's sweet sixteen it was crying with you about what happened. You cried because you actually cared, and you knew exactly how I would feel the next morning. Greg always told me you were his favorite of my friends, and it's not hard to see why. On a different note, not many people can still say they've remained best friends since the second grade, but we can. What have we not been through together? I'm pretty sure nearly every sporting event we ever participated in was with each other. I'm not even entirely sure we could have gotten through track season without each other. Pretty funny how we went from actually despising track to somewhat loving it AND loving soccer to kinda hating it within a two year time frame. But even though are [sic] mindsets and future plans significantly changed, our friendship has not. Can't believe we

actually ended up going to both of our dream colleges…
it's pretty awesome I gotta admit. The past couple years
have brought us closer than ever, and I honestly don't
know what I'll do without the sophwhores next year, but I'm
100 percent positive we will all stay best friends. It's amazing how much we have grown and matured these past
couple years. Going into high school I had no real idea of
who I'd be best friends with when I graduated, but I'm glad
it's you, because I know you are a lifelong friend. I know I
can ask you anything and you'll give me an honest opinion, and that's probably what I respect and admire most
about you. You are always real and genuine, and I hope
that never changes, because finding a person like that is
rare. F FAKE PEOPLE YES F THEM, those are the type
of people we dislike most. I cannot wait to visit each other
in college, where we will hopefully meet our future hus-
bands (crossing my fingers).

On the afternoon of December 28, Emma and Madison
went for a run, then to the Garden State Mall to shop for
outfits for New Year's Eve. The two friends were walking
past Urban Outfitters, toward Forever 21, and were considering what kinds of dresses they should buy for the upcoming
night. Part of their friendship centered on common interests,
on the hundreds of hours spent playing soccer and running
track, but their compatibility went beyond simple proximity.

The driving force was really how they complemented each other away from sports. Emma was steady, dependable, a pillar against which Maddy would occasionally lean, while Emma loved how lively Madison could be, how she often forced Emma to step outside her comfort zone.

So if Maddy was going to be able to tell any friend how she was really feeling, and maybe have that friend actually understand, Emma was that person. Maddy had already tried—kind of. She had texted Emma frequently about how unhappy she was at Penn, but Maddy also knew she hadn't given Emma much of a chance to help, hadn't peeled back the layers for her best friend. Madison had certainly never mentioned suicide. She wasn't sure she could say that word out loud, at least not to Emma, or to any of her other friends. But why couldn't she? Was it because the possibility was outlandish, seemingly dramatic and hyperbolic? Or was it because it was actually none of those things, and she didn't want anyone barricading the exit door she had pried open?

As the two walked between stores, Emma listened as Maddy talked to her about how bad things had gotten at school. "I keep Googling my symptoms because I don't really know what's going on, why I feel this way," she said.

"Feel what way?" asked Emma.

"I can't sleep. I wake up sweating. It's really hard for me."

"So what do you think it is?"

"Every time I Google it, it says it's just the adjustment to college," Maddy said.

"You don't think that's it?"

"It's just such a blanket answer—how could that be it? I'm down and sad all the time. I'm tired, but I can't sleep."

"But think about Ashley's experience during her freshman year, or my brother's when he went to college. This happens. People get sad. Right?"

"I know," Maddy said. "It just feels like what they were sad about is nothing like what I'm sad about."

"I was sad when I broke up with [my boyfriend]," Emma tried.

"I know," Maddy said. "When I've broken up with guys, it sucked. But this isn't like that."

"Okay."

"It's hard, not having answers," Maddy said. "I just want to know what's happening to me."

Madison had always had the answer, because finding the right answer had never been tricky, had never been an enigma, but rather was simply a matter of hard work. She was good at showing up and chipping away. But solving this problem was nothing like that. This was slippery, painful, and the harder she tried to understand what was happening, the worse she felt. The rules for this game were inverted, leaving her no clue how to play.

The two friends walked into Forever 21 and began looking through the racks. They each chose numerous dresses to try on, then walked back to the fitting rooms. Emma walked into one, Madison into the next. Changing topics, they started talking about New Year's Eve, about who would be at the party, about whether or not their high school boyfriends would be there, and if so, what might happen with them. She had seen a few guys down in Philly, but none had become exclusive relationships. But all that rational thinking would probably go out the window on New Year's Eve, when Maddy and Emma would start drinking in the early evening and, like most kids, likely make different, less sound decisions after midnight.

Each slipped into a new dress, tags still on, then stepped out to show the other. Emma's dress clung to her, and she watched as Maddy stepped into the hallway between the two fitting rooms. Maddy's dress was bunching in places, sagging in others, as if she were a young girl playing dress-up in her mom's clothes. Yet she hadn't chosen the wrong size; she had grabbed dresses in the size 4 she had always worn in high school. Emma didn't mention it.

The two kept slipping into other dresses, then stepping out to show each other, and eventually each settled on one, though Emma thought the outfit Madison chose was still too big on her. When Emma dropped off Maddy an hour later, she couldn't stop thinking about what her friend had been trying to tell her as they walked between stores. She pulled out her iPhone to send Maddy a message and noticed that her friend had already messaged her.

Madison: Currently with Trisha venting about my life haha idk what to do

Emma: I know I thought more about it once I dropped you off

Emma: I wanna talk about it more but the mall was not a good setting

Madison: Yeah we need to

Emma: Ya agreed

Madison: And what do ya think?

Emma: I know it's a tough position but I really think you should stick out the year at upenn and then decide

Madison: I'm just so stuck about it all.

Emma: I know that's not what you want to hear but I really think that's the best idea

Madison: And quit track? I fucking
hate it

Emma: Like so much you don't think
you could finish out the year?

Madison: I have zero fun/enjoyment
doing it at this point

Madison: legit.

On New Year's Eve everyone went over to Emma's to get
ready: Maddy, Justine, Jackie, Erin. The plan was to go to a
party at the house of a girl from their class at Northern Highlands. Madison had brought with her the dress from Forever
21. She put on the outfit and suddenly realized it didn't fit at
all. Her friends looked at her. "Maddy, how are you so
skinny?" they asked. "I don't know," she said finally. She
began looking through Emma's closet for something else to
wear. Eventually, after trying on a number of dresses and
finding that none fit, she grabbed a skirt, size 0, that managed
to stay just above her hips.

Madison had been particular about food for years. And
how could she not be? She was an athlete, a runner, and even
during high school, when she went out to dinner with her
family, she would order a salad while her parents and siblings
ordered burgers and fries. They came to accept this about

her, though Ashley would occasionally dangle a piece of pizza in front of her sister's nose and taunt, "Come on, you know you want some." Still, Maddy rarely ate anything that wasn't proper fuel for running—except when she was drunk. Then she would occasionally eat pizza, having clouded the part of her mind that policed food intake. Whenever this happened, she'd wake up early the next morning and go running, a kind of double penance for indulgence.

She especially liked peanut butter, and during her freshman year at Penn, she wrote a paper about her favorite food for an Intro Sociology class:

Some things never change. My favorite food, for example, has remained the same for as long as I can remember. Like many Americans, I grew up eating peanut butter and jelly sandwiches on a regular basis. Although my diet has expanded largely over the years and I am more willing to try new and diverse foods, something within me always brings me back to this one sandwich. It offers an instantaneous regression to my childhood. Although the employees at The Bridge Café on the University of Pennsylvania campus often give me a strange look when I place my order, nothing hinders my daily desire for the simplicity of a peanut butter and jelly sandwich...

The various social factors that have had a large influence on shaping my food practices are my family, our demographic background, and our financial and economic status. My hometown, Allendale, is a very affluent and costly town in northern New Jersey with high-class education and high taxes. In addition to this, I grew up living with four other siblings. My parents could not afford to provide money for each of us to individually buy lunch at school everyday. Faced with this challenge, my siblings and I resorted to peanut butter and jelly sandwiches as an affordable, simple and satisfying lunch.

For the past five to six years I set my own boundaries regarding the nutrition value of my foods because of my devotion to running. As a serious and competitive track athlete, I stay on a fairly regimented diet composed of fruits, vegetables, chicken, fish, granola bars, protein bars, and of course peanut butter and jelly sandwiches. However, the more popular and well-known brands of peanut butter such as Skippy, Jiff, and Peter Pan are not particularly "healthy." During my childhood I did not necessarily care about the brand because I was not too concerned with nutrition, but now health plays a vital part of my life since my performance in track depends in large part on my eating habits. Now I only eat organic, all natural peanut butter. As a good source of protein, carbs, and healthy fats, athletes such as myself commonly indulge in the peanut butter and jelly sandwich because of its healthy attributes.

Madison was particular about what she put in her body. However, that Christmas break, she did very little in moderation. The shift was slight, and easily explained—that is, if anyone was trying to explain it, which they weren't. Over break, Maddy wanted her good friends close, just the small group of them. Drinking excessively during winter break is hardly unusual behavior among teenagers and college students. In some ways, the more unusual occurrence would be a young person who has already mastered the art of moderation. When she went to the gym, often with Brooke, Madison would push herself harder than anyone else. During one workout Brooke looked over at her friend, who was on the bike, and thought it looked as if Maddy was trying to sweat something out of her body. She looked ferocious, desperate. Her head was down, sweat was pouring from her temples, her legs pumping as if on the final stretch of an uphill sprint. *What was motivating her in that moment?* Brooke wondered. But then she stopped wondering. She and Maddy had been close during high school, but they were the kind of friends who goofed off and laughed together, everything light and easy. Except for soccer, of course—that had always been serious for both of them.

Brooke,

I know that a handwritten letter is more personal, but you KNOW how bad my handwriting is, and when you read this again 10 years from now, I want you to actually be able to read what I wrote. You may make me laugh more than anyone else I know, and I know you are smiling right now about me admitting that. I know how much you enjoy when I laugh at your jokes (even if they aren't really all THAT funny). I will definitely miss your corny jokes and silly personality. And most of all, I will miss the amazing friend that you are to me. Brooke, if there is one person I know I can always count on for anything, it's you. You are kind-hearted, caring, compassionate, and trustworthy; all valuable characteristics of a friend that any girl would be lucky to have. When someone is upset or something goes wrong in any situation, you are always first to the rescue. Your selflessness is so admirable, but don't forget it is necessary to put yourself first sometimes. We still have so much room to grow and mature but I am so happy to say that you have played a huge role in the person I have become today.

I will never forget all the crazy times we spent together starting in the third grade on the Americans. Ever since that young age, I knew I could count on you 100 percent, whether it be in the goal and on the field or just in everyday situations. When it comes to soccer, you are the most determined and team-oriented person. Without you on the field/in goal, we would not have had the same amazing success. You've grown so much as a player and I expect big things from you at Holy Cross. I cannot wait to come watch you and Claire play. Ever since you were little, you've always been fearless and courageous, and you've only become stronger and braver over the years. If you ever need someone to shoot on you, I'm still your girl ☺ I loved warming you up before every NHGS game. And who knew that those warm-ups would lead to 48 WINS IN A ROW!?!?!?!?! Together, we've created a legacy at Highlands, and we should be damn proud of it. You were the starting goalie for a 2 year undefeated state championship team. That is freaking awesome. I would also like to award you as the most frequent Netflix viewer to ever live— hahahaha I know that will piss you off. Also when you read this in 15 years I wonder if you'll still be obsessed with your iPad...hahahahahaaa love you. Even though Madigan definitely doubted us at first, we exceeded her expectations and surprised everyone this season. There is no better feeling than playing and winning games with my absolute best friends. I know how much NHGS has always meant to you, and your obvious passion and love for the team quickly rubbed off on everyone else. It was contagious, and we can all attribute your passion as one of the reasons why we were so successful the past two seasons. I will never forget your absolutely amazing pasta parties.

What food DIDN'T Sharon make?!? She is legitimately bomb. And I will miss little Nicholas and Bridget and Richie. I cannot wait to see what they'll grow up to become when they are older. Tell Bridget she can go to any very smart school besides Harvard. Harvard sucks. And hopefully Richie can pull the Highlands Football team together... hahaha that'd be a miracle.

There is no one I'd rather spend gym class and health class with. How I met your mother??? Yes, you are obsessed. Can't believe you watched every single episode every season. Hahaaaaha you really do crack me up. Silly Brookie.

I know friends tend to drift apart after high school, but I hope that never happens to us. IM TRYNA BE FRIENDS FOR LIFE OK!!!! That is, if we both survive college. I have confidence that we will...well, you will. ☺ I hope you know how much I care for you and that I will always be here for you no matter what. You already had an incredible high school career and you'll only be more amazing in college.

Another reason Maddy's friends weren't concerned about her appearance over break: she had started losing weight before she left for Penn, so the change wasn't drastic. It wasn't as if Maddy had left for college looking one way and returned another; the progression seemed steadier, less easy to identify as a red flag.

During track season in her senior year, Maddy was particularly focused on her diet, because now she knew she would be running track in college. Running was a different beast than soccer, a spectacular balancing act. A runner is always attempting to control everything—time, energy, form, workouts, food intake, hydration—yet simultaneously conscious that she shouldn't become controlled by any one variable. She is the agent. It's as if each discipline is a necklace, and a runner must know when to put one on, when to take one off, when she can handle more than one, when she can't. If runners lose this talent for calibration, they end up wearing all the necklaces at once, and they sink. In other words, the art of elite running is often about the negative space. It's less about knowing when to run; more about knowing when not to.

At a track meet during senior year, a local photographer came up to the parents of one of Maddy's friends and asked about Maddy. For years, this woman had snapped pictures of Madison at Northern Highlands meets. She had a daughter who had run in college and who struggled with an eating disorder. That day, as she followed Madison inside the small black circle of the lens, with all outside influences closed off, she noticed a difference in the young woman she had spent hours watching. "I cannot believe the change in Madison," she said. "Crap—she got skinny."

No evidence exists, besides conjecture, to suggest that Maddy had an eating disorder. But plenty exists to suggest that she was, even before she left for Penn, attempting to control the uncontrollable. She wanted to hold water.

CHAPTER 7

Snow Falling

Madison was in her version of pajamas: a T-shirt and sweatpants. Emma wore a variation of the same, but with the Boston College logo instead of Penn's on the shirt. They had bagels and tea, and were making pancakes at Emma's house. The falling snow outside gave them a reason to stay hunkered down and to be lazy. A group of them had slept over at the Sullivans' house the previous night, including Brooke and Justine, but the other girls had to leave early, so it was Maddy and Emma, along with Emma's mom, Lorraine, who lingered in the kitchen, making breakfast and talking. It was Christmas break, so nobody had anyplace they had to be.

It was during these one-on-one interactions when Lorraine best understood her daughter's closest friend, though Lorraine was convinced that she might never truly connect with Maddy. A part of Maddy seemed closed off, unknowable. Oddly this tendency was exacerbated in group settings, when Madison would often retreat into herself, choosing to sit at the table and study rather than join everyone else. None of Madison's group noticed these subtle differences between their friend and everyone else, but how could they? They were immersed in these moments themselves. Their parents were of course less so. In addition, there was the simple matter of sample size and experience—their ability to place Maddy in a larger context, just one among thousands of other interactions. Having interacted with dozens of their kids' friends, the parents had a spectrum on which to judge the normalcy of each interaction, each person.

Emma saw Maddy from up close, as if looking in a mirror, while her parents and other adults were able to watch them both from afar, able to interpret the totality of their words and actions. "Madison is different than your other friends," more than one parent told a daughter during high school.

Lorraine was a good five years older than Maddy's parents, Jim and Stacy, but they had all grown up together on Long Island. The Holleran clan had been a big family around town. Although they had grown up in the shadows of New York City, the Long Island community operated almost like the small town Allendale was years later: people knew plenty about their neighbors. Depression and anxiety existed on

Jim's side of the family, but these weren't the types of issues that families often spoke about with one another or anyone else. Mental health issues were handled privately; things weren't spilled out into the open to be deconstructed and understood.

Madison, unfortunately, was never good at understanding why she was feeling a certain way. Often she communicated best through writing, not conversation. This made discussing her feelings with her parents and friends—beyond texting—very difficult.

Her demeanor in the kitchen at Emma's house was Exhibit A: she could not, or chose not to, name exactly what was happening with her at Penn. On this snowy morning in early January, the two friends openly expressed their shared disappointment with college. But after a while, the conversation tilted again toward Madison.

"So what exactly are you most upset about?" Lorraine asked.

"I think it's track," Maddy said. "It's making me unhappy—it's just too much. It's just not what I expected."

That felt like a problem Maddy could solve: stop running track.

"But it's more than that," she continued. "I'm spending so much time studying, but I can't seem to get ahead. And I'm tired all the time, but I can't sleep. And...I just don't know what exactly is wrong."

She was skinny, drained. So beautiful you couldn't stop

staring, and yet in that moment all you could notice was the emptiness in her eyes. She was twitchy, nervous, but didn't exactly know why. The conversation kept going in circles, with Emma and her mom trying to understand and help but Maddy failing to express anything tangible enough for them to untangle. Maddy would drop her head, clearly defeated, the gesture a kind of desperation conveying urgency, and this would launch them into another round of questions. This went on for hours.

At one point Lorraine considered asking her daughter's friend if suicidal thoughts had crossed her mind, but she dismissed the question as an extreme reaction. Maddy hadn't taken the conversation to that level and didn't seem to warrant that kind of concern, so Lorraine didn't want to hit a panic button that didn't exist. This question, to nearly everyone who considers it, feels loaded. They feel they may be introducing an option rather than reflecting one that's already been considered.

That morning, the conversation among the three of them continually circled back to one potential fix: Madison should quit track. She had, it seemed, hung her hopes on this solution. For the previous few weeks, Madison had been texting most of her friends, especially those from Northern Highlands, that she was considering quitting track or transferring, or occasionally both: quit track at Penn, then transfer to Lehigh to play soccer, or transfer to Vanderbilt, or, well— anything other than continuing with her current situation.

12/4/13 6:51 PM

Maddy: Like I wanna go to Lehigh now.

Emma: You would transfer???

Maddy: Idk

Maddy: Yeah

Maddy: I don't fucking know what to do

Maddy: Don't tell anyone this tho

Emma: Obviously not

Emma: But I don't know if you would wanna play for the Lehigh guy

Maddy: Idk but Clara loves it there

12/30/13 1:20 PM

Maddy: Would it be crazy if I transferred?? Lol

Izzy: Where?

Maddy: Idk I think maybe Vanderbilt

Maddy: Just for school

Maddy: F track

Maddy: I want to soooo badly

Maddy: I hate it

12/28/13 11:01 PM

Maddy: Not even kidding Ingrid I'm highly debating quitting too. Legit. So sad but I just don't like it at all anymore 😞

Ingrid: Me neither in fact I dread it

Maddy: My coach would be APPALLED. But like I seriously just wanna do club soccer

Maddy: What did your parents say?

Ingrid: My mom is totally supportive and my dad would be kinda disappointed that I didn't stick out a commitment

Ingrid: Have you talked to your fam about it?

> **Maddy:** Not exactly . . . but I need to ASAP. It would just make life so much easier but the concept of quitting is muuuuuuuch easier than carrying out the process haha like I don't even know how I would do it/what to say

12/28/13 11:03 PM

> **Maddy:** I may quit track 😳

Jack: Why . . .

Jack: You would be a NARP [non-athletic regular person]

> **Maddy:** I know which would fucking blow
>
> **Maddy:** But it SUCKS a lot

12/30/13

> **Maddy:** Emma I miss soccer and being on a CLOSE team

Maddy: Like I stalked Clara's Facebook and Lehigh looks so fun

Emma: I know . . . .

Emma: So much . . . .

Maddy: It fucking sucks idk what to do

Maddy: Like I wanna play again

Maddy: I'm so over my team in all honesty

Emma: Madison you can walk on . . . . .

Maddy: At Penn!? No fuckin way

Emma: Yessssss you are 100% good enough. The PENN STATE coach liked you

From: Madison Holleran
Date: Tue, Dec 31, 2013 at 9:46 AM
Subject: blood tests
To: REDACTED

Hi coach! Happy new years eve!!

Unfortunately, I won't be getting the results from the blood tests back until January 10th when I go back to the doctor. [Madison had blood tests to make sure she wasn't sick.] What should the plan be until then?

1/2/14

Emma: So Vanderbilt?

Maddy: I wanna!!!!!!

Emma: Ahhhhhhh!!!

Emma: Are you gonna go back?

Maddy: I don't wanna at all

Maddy: At all.

After cycling through all the options, ping-ponging from one to another over winter break, Madison seemed resigned to the fact that she would return to Penn for the second semester. She had been so thrilled with the Ivy League just months before: wouldn't it be a mistake to throw all that away? Her parents were doing the best they could, trying to shepherd their ailing daughter toward the best possible solution. They worried: Wouldn't she regret giving up on her dream so quickly? They didn't want to just throw open the doors and let her trample on her future. They wanted to help Maddy alleviate anxiety in a way that wouldn't set her back too far. Because the truth is, when you don't know the stakes, when you don't know how high the wire actually is, dancing along the edge doesn't seem reckless; it seems like the only place to walk.

By the time Maddy was sitting across from Emma and Lorraine, the question really wasn't whether she would return to Penn, but rather how she could improve her life there. Over the previous twenty-four hours, she had begun soliciting advice from her friends. She would soon begin to compose a letter to Steve Dolan, the Penn track coach, and she wanted help with the language and ideas; but mostly, she wanted her friends to participate, because then it would feel less like she was quitting. That afternoon, after spending the morning at the Sullivans', Maddy texted her teammate Ashley Montgomery.

1/3/14 2:14 PM

> **Maddy:** Ash I need to talk to you ☹️ ☹️

Ash: About what've

Ash: *what??

> **Maddy:** About track. Like I've honestly been thinking seriously about

transferring because I can't do it anymore. I'm going to talk to my parents about quitting track and seeing if things get better, but I just don't want the team to HATE me. Like completely hate me, but I just can't be happy doing it anymore like at all. It's awful. And I wish I could want to do it, but I can't. And I'm just completely stuck about it all.

Ash: They won't hate you you've gotta do what's right for you . . . is it a for sure decision and then you're gonna think about the transfer thing throughout the semester?

Maddy: No I don't WANT to transfer. I'm gonna see how this semester turns out ya know?

Maddy: Transferring just would be so complex and difficult

Maddy: I wanna love penn! Like we always said

Maddy: And I feel like that's possible to do

Maddy: Just gotta do the things that will make me happy again

Ash: Yeah well that makes sense are you gonna tell [Coach] Martin when you get back?

Maddy: Idkk yet gotta discuss with my mother and father first

On January 5, Ingrid texted Madison the link to an article on *The Huffington Post* titled "Ivy League Quitters: The Costs of Being an Ivy Athlete." The author, Jennie Shulkin, attended Penn. She wrote, "The abnormality of the varsity athlete's college experience begins even before he or she moves into the freshman dorms. Most Ivy athletes are officially recruited; they are accepted to the university in return for an informal agreement to serve on a sports team until graduation. This may sound like a good deal for the recruits, but it presently appears that the benefits of staying on an Ivy team are often not sufficient to prevent them from violating this informal agreement and quitting their respective sports."

Shulkin continued: "Ex-Penn athletes leave their teams for a lot of the same reasons. First, understand that unlike other NCAA Division I recruits, no Ivy League athletes are given athletic scholarships, and are therefore devoting their time and effort to a cause without the expectation of compensation. If an athlete quits, no money can be revoked (since none was given originally), and he or she is allowed to continue college without financial or educational consequences. That being said, roughly all recruits plan to honor their commitments. They want to be student-athletes.

"However, since athletes cannot be punished for reneging on their informal commitments, many of them feel compelled to quit when they realize that many of the costs simply outweigh the benefits."

The article went on to outline five key factors: the time commitment, the fact that sports seem to be the only priority of the coaches, the lack of reward or appreciation from others, the potential minimization of injuries, and the extra little things that push athletes over the edge. "The combination of the academics and athletics leaves little time for an internship or a part time job to earn extra income, an active social life, Greek life, clubs, and other aspects of a 'normal' college experience," Shulkin wrote.

1/5/14 9:05 PM

Ingrid: . . .

Ingrid: Published today. Maybe a sign?

Maddy: Hell yes

Maddy: Wait that article is SPOT ON

Ingrid: I know how crazy!!

Maddy: holy shit

Maddy: It's so true too

Ingrid: What did your mom say?

Maddy: It's definitely though like when I come back to penn I am 100 percent talking to my coach. Even with my mom like she's coming hahaha I can't do it anymore

Maddy: She really does not support the fact that I wouldn't be on a team or doing a sport because sports have always been a huge part of me but I told her that I'm gonna try out for club soccer next year. Also she knew that I really really wasn't happy on the team so she was like whatever will make you happiest, because she also knows that I really haven't been feeling Penn overall. So we both agreed that something has to change ya know?

Maddy: Because if track was one of the primary factors for making me unhappy then obviously that's gotta change.

Madison had kept her high school friends close the entire winter break. And on the night before the first among them would return for second semester, the group met at Justine's house for a potluck dinner. They called this potluck "The Last Supper," because so many of them were dreading the return to school. Each was responsible for bringing one item. Usually, Maddy would bake. She loved making cookies, often peanut butter ones. Throughout high school she would make homemade cookies for people—baking was a hobby of hers, even if eating the cookies was not.

That night, Madison brought cookies from Pathmark, which she arranged nicely on a platter. The group of friends sipped wine and reminisced about high school and discussed how surprisingly difficult college had been. When dessert time came, Madison pulled out the tray of Pathmark cookies.

But MJ had made a homemade variation of s'mores. Next to this effort, Maddy's cookies looked lackluster. Not to be deterred, she began breaking the cookies in half and placing them on everyone's plates.

"You think if you break them up, it's going to look like people want them?" joked Brooke, whose relationship with Maddy had always been one of needling each other. Brooke began collecting all the broken cookies, piecing them back together, then returning them to the Pathmark container, proving that none had been eaten. Maddy laughed.

During the dinner, Madison sent a text message to Ingrid that included a picture of the seven friends, arms around one another. "These are the types of friends we need to find at Penn," she wrote beneath the image. At the end of the night, everyone hugged. Madison kept repeating, "Love you, see you soon!" as if their future held endless nights like these.

Maddy had told all her friends, even those she wasn't especially close to, that she planned to quit track. And, as she and her parents had discussed, she had sent an e-mail to Steve Dolan requesting a meeting once she had returned to campus. Stacy was planning to drive down to Philadelphia to join her daughter for the sit-down. Dolan responded to the e-mail the afternoon before Maddy returned to school.

On Fri, Jan 10, 2014 at 2:29 PM, Stephen Dolan wrote:

Madison,

I'm looking forward to seeing you and talking on Monday. Congratulations on such a strong first semester academically. Just so you know, you had the 5th highest semester GPA of our entire women's track team!

See you soon!

From: Madison Holleran
Date: Fri, Jan 10, 2014 at 9:53 PM
Subject: Re: Penn Track
To: Stephen Dolan

Thanks! Certainly wasn't an easy semester. Looking forward to seeing you too!

1/10/14 3:26 PM

Greg: What's going on with everything? Are you going back to school? Are you running track?

Greg: Hahaha sorry for the overload. If you don't want to talk about it idc.

Maddy: Hahahahahaa

Maddy: Yes I'm going back to school tomorrow. Can't say I'm ecstatic. And I'm having a meeting with my coach about everything on Monday. And as of now, not anticipating to stay on track

Greg: 😞 das mah face. I guess you gotta do what's best for you though. It makes me a little sad to think about you not playing a sport. Tomorrow though?!!!! No coffee ☕ 😨. I guess that just means a trip to Penn is in order!!

1/10/14 2:54 PM

Maddy: Going back to skewl tomorrow ✌️

Will: Just saw that text from last night 😨

Maddy: 😨 🙈 🙈 🙈

Maddy: Imma give Penn another shot

Maddy: 1 more chance

Will: It's like a slap in the face cause penn is so much more fun than Princeton

Will: I feelz ya

Maddy: Yeah it is really fun hahah I just don't know if it's the right school for me yaaaa know

Maddy: penn rocks my socks

Maddy: im determined to like this semester

Will: _100_

Maddy: 🐺 🐧

Madison Holleran
Writ015-302 Medieval in Art and Film
Final Portfolio
Cover Letter
3 December 2013

Dear reader,

My decision to take writing seminar during the first semester of college is something I most certainly do not regret. In all honesty, because of the "Medieval in Art and Film" seminar and the "known-item outline" assignment, I checked out the first book of my college career from Van Pelt library...As the semester comes to an end, I can proudly say I look forward to utilizing my newly acquired skills from this course in the many other courses I will take part in at Penn.

Thank you,

Madison Holleran

In high school, Maddy's favorite teacher had been Mr. Quinn, who taught math. She liked the subject, and she liked the way Mr. Quinn taught, but she actually preferred writing. Even though she was drawn to the arts, she was concerned about pursuing it as a degree or as her future career. Business school, she thought, would be a much more direct, reasonable path. She mentioned to Emma that perhaps she would try transferring to Wharton, Penn's famed business school. "Really, she was confused as to what she wanted to do," Emma said. "She honestly didn't know. She liked writing, and I remember her saying maybe she could be a writer later on. But she knew it was hard to graduate from college and write. 'If I go to business school,' she told me, 'that would be more practical.' I think I could see her in communications, in public relations, for sure—something with fashion or social media. I know she would be smart enough for business, but she didn't love it."

Maddy's imagination, her free spirit, kept snagging on the hook of practicality.

The Quitting Game

When I wanted to quit basketball during my freshman year at the University of Colorado, I told my friends and roommates my plan, which was both a way of testing the idea and also a way of gauging my ability to say the words aloud. Quitting sounded weak. But also delicious and necessary, and I vacillated between desperately wanting to never again dribble a basketball and also fearing that I was nobody without the sport.

None of my friends and roommates told me not to quit. After barely a pause, they all said something like "Whatever will make you happy," then went about their day. I didn't quite understand at the time that very few people (save for a parent, maybe a best friend) spend much time thinking about someone else's problems. Asking for permission rarely results in layered, nuanced discussion. And even if it had, I had no clue how I might explain myself because I really didn't know what I wanted; I just knew something needed to change.

I was terrified of the word "quit." Within sports, that word is dirty and barely distinguishable from "I can't." I had come to view quitting as synonymous with laziness, weakness, and selfishness. If you quit during a drill, you were lazy and weak. If you quit in the middle of a season, maybe you were not only lazy and weak, but selfish, too, willing to let down your teammates. Strict parameters like this felt suffocating, impossible to navigate, as if everywhere I turned, the door to leaving was slamming closed. If I tried to push out anyway, everyone watching me leave would also be judging me. Could I ever stop? Could something be too much without me being not enough? The either/or thinking that permeates sports makes stepping aside, during a drill or a season, a referendum on character, on its deficiencies.

What was the difference between quitting and stopping, or quitting and retiring, or quitting and making the conscious decision that continuing something was genuinely unhealthy? The difference lay in semantics. And yet, depending on the lens through which someone else viewed my decision (which I could not control), I would become in their eyes either wise or weak—and more likely the latter. Of this, I was keenly aware. (So, too, was Madison.)

How much of our happiness is fueled by society's validation of our choices? It seems that the younger we are, the more dependent we are on making choices others will value and praise—perhaps because we haven't developed, or don't yet fully trust, our ability to name or even know what makes us happy.

In my memoir, *The Reappearing Act,* I told a version of the following story (with some expanded thoughts added below) about my attempt to quit college basketball:

> I did not want to play basketball anymore; could not stand another day of practice. And that's exactly what I was about to tell Ceal Barry, the head women's basketball coach at Colorado, the woman who had believed in me enough to offer a full scholarship. She was not the only coach to recruit me, but she was the only one whose program was consistently nationally ranked. When it came down to deciding where to go to school, I chose CU because I wanted to test myself at the highest level athletically. And here I was, crumbling beneath the weight—after only a few weeks of official basketball practice. I became desperate for everyday moments, which felt exotic. A trip to the grocery store made me feel like an outsider. Walking the aisles, watching people fill their carts, I felt as if I was in the zoo, on the outside looking in. I yearned to go home after classes and cook, to see movies, to do all the things I saw those around me doing, but which I never had time for. I became resentful.

That day I met Coach Barry, I was still wearing my practice gear: black mesh shorts and a reversible mesh jersey. I had grabbed my sweatshirt from the cubicle inside the weight room and pulled it over my head. Coach Barry was walking in front of me, leading the way out of the weight room, then snaking through the training room and into a corner office of some assistant trainer who wasn't at work because it was Saturday. She flipped on the lights and lowered herself into the office's chair.

My teammates and I had just lifted weights inside the Dal Ward Athletic Center, which overlooked the football stadium and offered, especially at dusk, an inspiring view of the Flatirons, the Boulder foothills leading to the crescendo of the Rocky Mountains. I stumbled my way through the lifting session, choking back tears, feeling broken, barely able to keep the dumbbells from crashing down and splitting my head open.

I slipped into the room with Coach Barry, but stood just inside the doorway, my back covering the light switch, as if I wasn't fully committed to being there. At that moment, I didn't feel capable of committing to much of anything. Coach didn't seem to have any inkling of what I might say, but she was definitely aware of how pathetic I had been at practice lately. I closed the door behind us. She looked at me, expectantly.

"I just…" I glanced at her, then down at the tops of my sneakers. I told myself to look up again, to be mature. I met her gaze. "I think I'm going to have to quit," I said. "That's all. That's what I needed to say."

She leaned forward, closing the distance between us, and let out a long breath. My commitment to quitting was strong, but not ironclad. Although I was a sophomore academically, I was in my freshman season with the basketball team because I had spent the previous year on the injured list, after being granted a medical redshirt. I was diagnosed with a stress fracture in my right foot during the fall of 1999, before basketball practice even started, and I eventually had season-ending surgery that December, with the team doctor inserting a screw into the bone to keep it from fully breaking. As a result, I spent my first year at CU hanging out with my teammates and getting all of the benefits of being a college athlete without having to do much of the serious training. The list of perks was long: status of being a college athlete, free gear, behind-the-scenes access to football games, meals at training table, and, most importantly, the emotional support and companionship of a team. The coaching staff redshirted me, which meant I retained that year of eligibility.

As I stood in front of Coach Barry that October day, I was healthy again, at least physically. I could run and jump and shoot; I just had zero motivation to do so.

I had convinced myself I didn't like basketball anymore. In fact, I took it one step further: I had *never* liked basketball. My father, Chris, was the one who loved the game; I was just mimicking him this entire time. And now that I was in the thick of it—hours and hours of mandatory practice, six days a week—I was being exposed as a fraud...

"I think quitting is a mistake," Coach Barry said, lifting her head. She seemed about to say more, but paused, perhaps wanting to see how I would respond. I leaned into the wall and bounced my shoulders a few times, looking at the ceiling.

"My heart is just not in it," I said, and I could feel my eyes burning, the twisting of the faucet behind my tear ducts. "I'm scared to death of practice. It's the last place in the world I want to be. Nothing is going right."

This last part was true; I was playing terribly. Coming out of high school, I had thought I was so damn good. I was one of the better scholastic players in New York State, but now I couldn't even finish a drill without being told I had done it the wrong way and needed to do it over—and why was I so pathetic? (The last question was my own addition, the kind of destructive self-talk I gave in to as I walked to the end of the line during drills.)

Coach Barry stood and took a step toward me. She half sat, half leaned on the desk, clasping her hands on her lap. "This is what we'll do," she said. "You'll give me two more weeks, and I'll change how I coach you. I think that's the problem here. Just give me two weeks."

My lack of perspective was frightening in that moment. To me, two weeks felt like an outrageous sentence handed down by an angry judge. We practiced six days a week in the preseason, sometimes twice a day. Two weeks meant twelve to fourteen practices, totaling about forty hours of basketball. And do you know how many drills can be packed into that amount of time?

In my young mind, time was distorted. Even now, years later, I can still feel how panicked I felt about a period of time—just two weeks—that, now, I would consider manageable for just about anything. And I can distinctly remember how those words—*fraud, weak, failure, quitter*—rattled like rocks around my brain.

In 2013, *The Guardian,* a British newspaper, published an

article under the headline "A stopwatch on the brain's perception of time: Research by neuro-physiologists shows that our emotions affect our awareness of the passing of time." In it, the paper dissects a study by French doctors who sought to understand how dopamine, which is usually lower in those dealing with depression, might affect our perception of time.

> Above all, the brain's perception of time involves processes linked to memory and attention: witness the impression that time is passing more quickly when we are busy, or doing something amusing or exciting. Time flies even when we are in love. In contrast, a watched pot never boils. Minutes drag by when we are bored...
> Dopamine is the main neurotransmitter involved in time processing. Dopamine agonists—compounds that activate dopamine receptors—tend to speed up our perception of time, which passes more quickly.
> Recent research by neuro-physiologists and chemists working on time processing is beginning to show how emotions may speed up or slow down our perception of time. In 2011 professor Droit-Volet and Sandrine Gil, a lecturer on cognition and learning at Poitiers University, France, published a study of how

changes in the emotional state of subjects caused by watching films affect their sense of time.

Two weeks of basketball practice. Two more weeks of track practice. Two weeks until a college counselor has an opening in their schedule. Two more months of first semester. Six more months of freshman year. Four more years of college. A lifetime of uncertainty.

In 2015, I thought of all these variables as I sat with a hundred students inside the journalism building on the University of Massachusetts campus. Sitting in that room with me were students of all genders, athletes and nonathletes, freshmen and seniors, black and white and brown. But when we arrived at the topic of pressure, of perfectionism and quitting, all of them reacted the same way: knowingly. They had felt these pressures, to varying degrees. And they seemed hungry to be understood, and hungry to hear that many of their peers had felt the same way.

Those lucky enough to grow up envisioning college start hearing about the building blocks of a college résumé (the boxes that need checking; the optics that need preserving) from the moment they enter high school, and sometimes even sooner. Too often, kids are herded into commitments and activities that are born not of passion but of obligation. These obligations can continue for years because stopping is not seen as a possibility. Those who do stop risk being perceived as lacking the intestinal fortitude to push through when the going gets tough.

Of course, sometimes (perhaps even often) inner strength is exactly what's needed and quitting is absolutely the wrong move, and if you push through the low points, you may find a reserve within yourself you never knew you had. But at other times, a commitment or decision can be accurately identified as the cause of unhappiness, and continuing to walk in that direction isn't necessarily going to lead you through the wilderness to a bright, blue clearing with birds chirping and a flowing river at your feet. Continuing that path can bury you deeper and deeper in the woods until you're lost, with no memory of how to get out.

Knowing the difference requires listening to and trusting yourself. Picture a doctor holding a stethoscope to your heart so that she can decipher even the shallowest of beats, the subtle shift in rhythm. That is the kind of precision with which you must know yourself in order to make these types of fork-in-the-road decisions. Yet are we equipping kids with the tools to pursue this empowering self-knowledge?

In *Excellent Sheep: The Miseducation of the American Elite*, William Deresiewicz observes that our education system seems to be producing kids who have trouble thinking critically and finding their purpose. In an interview with *Slate,* he offered the following insight: "The point is not what you do but why you do it, how you choose it...I understand that parents are worried about their children's future. But we have to look at what we're doing to our kids. We have to have the strength to raise them to care about something other than 'success' in the very narrow terms in which it's come to be defined. I'm not saying you can have it all: In fact, that's one of my biggest messages in the book. You have to choose. Parents already tell their kids to 'do what you love' and 'follow your dreams.' But kids know that they don't really mean it, that what they really want is status and success. Well, we have to really mean it."

Inside that room at the University of Massachusetts, I told the story of how I had tried to quit college basketball. Yet before I got to my ultimate point, I looked out at the audience and could almost see their eyes glazing over, bracing to be scolded—perhaps about the frequency of quitting among their generation, about their collective lack of follow-through and focus. But that wasn't my point at all. In fact, it was the opposite: Didn't they agree that the stigma around quitting sometimes forces us to stay in toxic situations? And wasn't it possible that this is even worse among millennials, who have been accused of being a fickle, lazy generation who require things to go their way?

At this the students seemed to lean forward, to let out a collective sigh. I asked whether any of them understood what I was trying to say—if they could relate, or if I was projecting my ideas onto the next generation. They stayed silent for a minute. Then a number of hands lifted. A young woman in the front row caught my eye. I nodded, encouraging her to share.

"I'm a sophomore now, here, but I initially started at a different college," she said. "I was so unhappy, right from the beginning, but I didn't think I could tell anyone, because I had told everyone that was the school of my dreams. I didn't want anyone to think I was giving up, or quitting. And I couldn't even understand, myself, if I was being weak, or if I genuinely needed to leave."

"Right?" I said. "Sometimes it's so confusing to know what the 'best' decision is—because, really, ultimately, who even knows?"

"I just got to a point where I was so unhappy, I talked to my parents about it."

"What did they say?"

"They were supportive, but of course they didn't want me to leave that school, because it was a brand name, and they were worried that I was jeopardizing my future options. And they were worried that I was too young to know what I wanted."

"And how did you feel?" I asked.

"Trapped—it just wasn't for me. And it finally got to the point where losing the identity of that school, how it supposedly reflected positively on me, was less important than needing to walk away and be happy again."

"How did your parents deal with that?"

"They get it now. They see how much calmer and happier I am here."

She lifted her UMass water bottle, took a sip. We continued the conversation for another half hour, the large group now beginning to resemble something more intimate. Some in attendance had transferred to UMass from other schools, while still others had considered leaving, perhaps believing they would be happier elsewhere. All were concerned about image—not just their own, but also the image of their generation as one that pursues self-satisfaction and happiness supposedly with brazen disregard for anything else, including ideals of responsibility and the greater good.

I took a leave of absence from ESPN to write parts of this book. On the first day I sat down to write, an e-mail popped into my inbox from Erik Rydholm, who is the executive producer of both *Around the Horn* and *Pardon the Interruption*. The note included an audio file as well as a few sentences: "I wanted to pass along this sermon by the late Maurice Boyd. He preached in NYC for decades before passing in 2005. Luckily, some 600 or so of his sermons were recorded. This one is probably my favorite, and when I was listening to it again this morning, it made me think of you and Madison and this book."

Boyd delivered this sermon, "The Fine Art of Being

Imperfect," in 1996. Apparently the Irish pastor never wrote out his sermons, but rather scribbled down a few notes and extrapolated on the ideas as he stood before his flock.

To make his point about the varying human responses to imperfection, Boyd uses three examples: Waterford crystal, pottery, and oriental rugs. At Waterford, Boyd explains, each piece of crystal is meticulously inspected, held up to the light, each surface appraised for the slightest crack or deformity. If any is spotted, the piece is immediately shattered. Boyd allows this imagery to sink in, allows the listener to picture the beautiful crystal being smashed against a hard object, the pieces swept away, punishment for a defect nearly invisible to the human eye. Then Boyd urges us to consider the slight space between these two wildly different outcomes. He says, "Notice how close perfection is to despair."

Then he moves on to pottery. As a potter's hands move over clay, shaping the malleable form, occasionally a mistake is made, an unwanted alteration to the vision. But usually the potter will not throw away the clay; she will attempt to reshape the piece around the mistake, as if it had never happened.

Then Boyd turns to the weavers who create the world's most beautiful rugs. They spend hours creating designs by hand, and during this painstaking process the shapes and angles often become lopsided, asymmetrical. However, this asymmetry is not considered a mistake to be eradicated or smoothed out. In fact, it is the opposite: this imperfection becomes the rug's beauty, its uniqueness. This rug is unlike any other, and that is what makes it a coveted work. Boyd's message asks a single question of his listeners: In which way do we view imperfection?

And, again: *Notice how close perfection is to despair.*

CHAPTER 8

The Meeting

Madison had returned to Penn two days early to see Jackie's first Ivy League game. But she also wanted to be on campus without obligations, to know what it felt like to walk through the streets, across the quad, without a grueling workout to get to—or even a class. Perhaps she would see Penn differently, fresher somehow. She wanted so badly for this semester to be different. She had made herself a promise: bring a different attitude to second semester.

That night, Maddy opened the notes application on her repaired iPhone and typed out her mantra:

new mindset

new everything

i can do this

i will do this

you CHOOSE your fate

willing to give it another chance

DON'T LOOK BACK

LOOK FORWARD

SETBACKS ARE NEEDED TO GET STRONGER

transferring is not an option

And if this forced positivity didn't work, somewhere on the back burner resided a different solution. But maybe Maddy wouldn't need that. Quitting track, she believed, would change everything, would be the jump start she needed to see the world differently. And not even drastically differently, just more like the way she had before, in high school.

She closed the notes application. She had said goodbye to her dad at the game, said goodbye to Ingrid a few hours later, after they'd watched the men play. Now she was back in her Penn dorm room—alone. It was nearly midnight on Saturday night.

She opened her MacBook, launched Pages, and began typing.

Although this has been extremely difficult to put into words, I'm going to do my best to explain my first semester at Penn and where it's led me.

Before I begin I just want to say I have the utmost respect and admiration for you as a coach and a person and that I know I wouldn't be at this school if it weren't for you. I also want you to know that you aren't at fault for anything negative I've felt over the past couple months in any way.

Here goes.

Yesterday was the first day since early September that I felt genuinely happy, that I actually felt like myself again, and that I felt like Penn MIGHT actually be the right place for me and that I felt excited to be here.

Yesterday was the first time since late October that I actually enjoyed running and really really wanted to run.

Yesterday was the first day in many, many months that I woke up feeling faithful and optimistic about my future since I knew I had reached a decision.

Maddy named the file "for dolan" and saved it to her Documents folder, alongside the papers she had written during first semester. In that folder there was also a document named "good quotes" to which she contributed whenever she stumbled upon a quote or poem she wanted to remember. The first entry on the page was from Helen Keller: "Life is either a daring adventure or nothing. Security does not exist in nature, nor do the children of men as a whole experience it. Avoiding danger is no safer in the long run than exposure." The next two on the page were similar, about how only those who leave home or get lost ever really find home or themselves. The final quote on the page was from Anne Frank: "Think of all the beauty still left around you and be happy."

In the Notes application on her iPhone, Maddy usually wrote down songs she wanted to remember. The list started in the summer of 2012 with "Dare You to Move" by Switchfoot. A week later she added "Still" by Matt Nathanson, and a few days after that, the song "Sort Of" by Ingrid Michaelson, followed by "I Will Follow You into the Dark" by Death Cab for Cutie. Maddy wrote down song titles throughout the summer of 2012, but then wrote nothing for sixteen months. Then, four months into her first semester at Penn, just before winter break, she again started listing song titles, but the sentiment behind these choices appears to have taken a drastic turn, from angst-filled love songs to something else entirely. On December 17, 2013, Maddy entered "Jesus Take the Wheel," and a day later she typed out "When I am lost, god is there," which wasn't a song title but rather a phrase she wanted to keep in mind.

As first semester wore on and her mind became more and more cluttered, Maddy had started going back to church.

Maddy was losing control, spending so many nights tossing and turning, so she returned to the one place that preached peace and calm. And over the holidays, she changed the bio on her Instagram to include verse Matthew 17:20. According to the New International Version of the Bible, the verse reads: "'You don't have enough faith,' Jesus told them. 'I tell you the truth, if you had faith even as small as a mustard seed, you could say to this mountain, 'Move from here to there,' and it would move. Nothing would be impossible."

That first night back in the dorm alone, Maddy reached for her phone and texted Emma.

> **Maddy:** HERES TO NEW BEGIN-NINGS THIS SEMESTER

> **Emma:** Seriously though. Totally different mind set!!

> **Maddy:** YES

> **Emma:** A no fucks given attitude

> **Maddy:** hahahahaah yes.

The upcoming meeting with Dolan was all Maddy could think of. She had never before quit anything, let alone her dream since she had started playing sports at age seven. The words needed to be perfect. She needed to show Coach Dolan the depth of her consideration, in the hope he would understand that she hadn't arrived at her decision lightly. Deciding to quit pained her deeply, more deeply than however that decision might affect anyone else in her life. But she had looked at this thing from all angles, and it was the necessary step. Maddy needed to convey that kind of urgency, to make the decision airtight, no loopholes. Because she didn't trust herself to speak with the same conviction with which she wrote, she kept writing and revising, and then writing more, until she felt she had achieved the right tone in her letter.

She did this on Sunday morning, again on Sunday night, and once more on Monday morning, the day Stacy and her sister Mackenzie would drive down to Philly and join her for the meeting with Dolan. Maddy had asked her mom if she could be there for support. Tapping on her MacBook, Maddy constructed sentence after sentence, carving out a letter that would detail what she believed was unavoidable: she needed to stop running.

In total, the past couple months have been an experience almost completely opposite from what I expected of college. For the most part, my experience at Penn so far has been a complete and total challenge. It's been a mental struggle which has led me to a place so low that I never ever thought was personally attainable. I never thought it was possible to sink so low, so drastically. I don't know how or when this all started, but everything seemed to get worse and worse as the first semester progressed. I've thought about leaving Penn for good. I've had difficulty sleeping, concentrating, making decisions, studying, and just overall have not been feeling like myself. Although I'm giving Penn a second chance, this semester made me very very unsure about whether or not it is the place for me. Through the daily routine of waking up and going to class, going back to my room and starting homework, going to practice then going to dinner and showering and heading to study hall, and coming straight back to my dorm to shower and do more homework before bed, the primary emotions I felt throughout the past couple months were overwhelmed, anxious, desperate and for the most part, lonely. Before coming to Penn I absolutely LOVED to run. After soccer practices ended in high school I would come home and run more just for the fun of it. Just because it served as sort of a mental therapy for me, a way to clear my mind and get a break from the daily responsibilities and obligations that life brings. Before coming to Penn I was beyond excited to run cross country because I have never done it before. I don't know where things went wrong, but ever since the middle of cross country season, my life seemed to be hurtling downwards and early on in the year I began to feel completely and utterly lost…as if I was in a whole other world and as if I no longer could recognize my purpose here, not my purpose as a part of the team, but my purpose in life. As hard as I tried to complete my workout packet over break, and as badly as I wanted to WANT to run, I just couldn't make myself do it. The running over the past couple months has taken a huge toll on me mentally, emotionally, and physically.

Writing this letter created in Maddy an emotion she hadn't recently felt: hope. She became increasingly convinced that quitting was the right decision. The hope began to gain momentum, a kind of high, and she started focusing on additional ways she could improve her quality of life during second semester. By Sunday night she was practically giddy with a mix of excitement and nerves.

From: Madison Holleran
Date: Sun, Jan 12, 2014 at 8:25 PM
Subject: open room?!—306 Thomas Penn?
To: REDACTED

Hi! I'm Madison Holleran, a freshman at Penn and I live in Hill College House. I am on the track team and I am currently rooming with one of my teammates. However, I have not been enjoying track at all recently and am planning on quitting the team very soon. I applied for a room change during the room switch period during first semester but did not end up getting a new room. One of my best friends just moved into 304 Thomas Penn and I noticed that there is an open room right next to her, 306 Thomas Penn. Is there any way I could move into that room?? Thanks, hope to hear back from you soon!

1/12/14 9:42 PM

Maddy: So nervous for tomorrow!!!!!!!!!!!!!!!!!!!!!!!!!!!!!!!

Emma: Talking to the coach???

Maddy: Ya betch

Emma: What time

Maddy: 11

Emma: Omg are you def gonna quit

Maddy: Attempting

Maddy: Lolz

Emma: OMG is Stacy coming

                               Maddy: Ya betch

Emma: I'm happy for you

Emma: And proud

                               Maddy: Ahahhaahahaaah I love u

1/12/14/ 9:40 PM

                               Maddy: Hi sweet mother of sweetness I'm doing well thanks!! Proud of Jackie and so happy I got to witness the first points of her college career 😊 she must have been so excited

Susie Reyneke: I hope you can stop putting so much silly pressure on yourself and just start enjoying your time there! I really liked your school!!

                               Maddy: Yeahh I know. Penn is a really fun and good place with a lot to offer, I just really don't enjoy track at all anymore.

Madison continued to write, to perfect the letter, working late into Sunday night, then again on Monday morning, as Stacy and Mackenzie made the drive south from Allendale to Philadelphia.

During high school after I made my decision to bail on Lehigh soccer and commit to Penn track, I was 100 percent sure it was the best decision I have ever made since my track times were peaking and I reached more success than I had ever thought was possible," she wrote. "After running the 1200 leg at Penn Relays I could not wait to compete for Penn. Then how did I end up here right now, wanting to leave the team and not competitively run anymore? How did I end up wanting to quit the team almost a month into school? How did I end up being as overall unhappy as I have been for the past four months? Before coming to Penn I was confident, focused, motivated, silly and mainly just a happy girl...

On Monday morning, Madison finished the letter. She printed out a copy, then sent a text to Ingrid and another of her friends at Penn, Alex:

1/13/14 10:32 AM

Maddy: Just finished the letter to my coach. 🙏 🙏 🙏 🙏 I'll update you guys when I get out of the meeting.

Alex: Good luck!! ☘

1/13/14 10:17 AM

Maddy: Meeting with my coach in 40 mins. HELLLPPPPP scared

Gabb: Good luck

As Stacy and Mackenzie arrived in Philly, they stopped at Starbucks and got Maddy her favorite, a vanilla latte, then drove to her dorm room, collected her, and the three of them went to the grocery store.

Although Mackenzie was confused about how Maddy could dislike college so much, she wasn't particularly worried. Mack had played a lot of sports while growing up and now also in high school, and she had wanted to quit before, so she could relate to how Maddy was feeling about running. She had been surprised at how distant and sad her sister had seemed over break. She remembered one night when the three sisters had been in Maddy's room, sitting on the bed, and that when Ashley left the room, tears started pouring down Madison's face.

"I'm not happy," she said, then kept repeating the same question: "How can I be happy? How...how?"

Mackenzie kept offering solutions: stop running, join a club, join a sorority, play soccer, go out more. "It's gonna change," Mack said. "It's gonna get better."

Now here they were in Philly, about to make the first of those changes. At the store they stocked up on healthy snacks for the fridge in Maddy's dorm room. They bought her baby carrots and hummus and organic peanut butter. There wasn't much time before the meeting with Dolan, so they quickly dropped off the groceries and all three went to the track offices. Maddy had her letter with her—two single-spaced pages— and she planned on reading the letter aloud to Coach Dolan.

Both terrified and thrilled by the statement she was holding, Maddy felt confident that the ideas she had expressed in the letter were urgent enough that Coach Dolan would understand why she had to make this change. Still, she needed to make absolutely clear to him, both in how she presented the letter and how she expressed her feelings, that no other choice existed. The meeting would change everything. She would no longer be the star athlete who could clear every hurdle, push through every obstacle. She would become Madison Holleran, student, normal in all the ways she had never been normal. The cost of this change would be high, but she had already run it by her friends and family, and although her identity seemed to be shifting dramatically, almost everyone had appeared to understand. And anyway, the truth was, the cost of staying inside her current identity—Madison Holleran, Ivy League runner—was steeper.

Maddy, Stacy, and Mackenzie walked into the athletic offices. While they waited in the lobby, Maddy showed the pages of the letter to her mom and sister, detailing the gist of what she wanted to say: she was unhappy; she needed to quit. When Coach Dolan appeared, waving them into a conference room, Maddy turned to her sister and said, "Can you stay here?"

"Oh, okay, yeah," Mack said. As her mom and sister went into the room, Mack found a chair. She pulled out her iPhone and began looking at prom dresses. The dance was still months away, but Mack had already started looking at options, and she would want her sister's input.

Mack wished she could be inside the conference room, mostly because she wanted to know specifically what Maddy's letter said. Nevertheless, she thought she understood what would happen behind the closed door: her sister would quit track. She knew that's what her sister wanted, and her sister had always been good at getting what she wanted.

Stacy remembers the conference room and its center table feeling big, but the three of them sat together in a corner. The coach wasn't sure what this meeting might hold, but over the years he'd had hundreds of similar meetings, listening as so many young athletes worked through the pressures of the college transition. Dolan led off the conversation by saying he didn't think Maddy was struggling as much as other athletes he had coached, and he thought she and Penn were a perfect match. From his vantage point, she had made one of the smoother transitions he had witnessed: She was in the team's top five on the cross-country course, she worked out great, she did well in school. In person, she seemed to be smiling, happy. And he hadn't heard differently from anyone—neither teammates nor coaches. "We saw this successful, well-liked person," Dolan said later. "It was fun to watch her excel and be excited."

The idea of burdening others, of dragging down her family and her teammates, appalled Maddy. The wilderness of her internal life, the constant waves threatening to overwhelm her, was her terrain—and hers alone—to navigate. In fact, the letter in her hands was more self-revelatory than she was used to being. But the change she hoped to spark was drastic, and she knew it required exposing more of herself than might be comfortable.

The three of them exchanged pleasantries. They spoke of winter break and holiday celebrations and rest, and how Maddy was feeling (the blood tests, which she and the coaches had e-mailed about in December, showed nothing alarming). Dolan shared with Maddy how well she had done first semester, how impressed with her he had been. None of this was particularly relevant to Maddy, but it was to Stacy, who hoped her daughter could hear the praise and reassurance, the validation. Couldn't she see? Her panic about first semester was a monster of her creation; she had given this monster life, and she could kill it, too.

Dolan circled back to the point of the meeting: how Maddy was feeling after first semester.

"I actually wrote a letter that I want to read," Maddy said, pulling out the two pages. "I wanted to make sure I said everything clearly."

She took a deep breath, then began: *"Although this has been extremely difficult to put into words, I'm going to do my best to explain my first semester at Penn and where it's led me..."*

Tears began spilling from Maddy's eyes, rolling down her cheeks. Stacy began crying, too, for very little in this world is more painful than seeing your child in pain. "I felt so bad for her," Stacy said. "I had never really seen her so distressed." Maddy continued reading the letter to her coach:

"How did I end up being as overall unhappy as I have been for the past four months? Before coming to Penn I was confident, focused, motivated, silly and mainly just a happy girl. But over the past couple months I've felt lost. And this feeling has accumulated and built up into so much more, and that's why I decided that something has to change. For as long as I can remember sports have defined me, but now I think it's time for another path. Now I think it's time to define myself. Thank you for giving me the opportunity to compete for Penn

and be a part of Penn track, but right now, I'm really not ready to compete. I don't know what is the right choice for me here at Penn, how to be 'happy' again, but I know something needs to change. And if I could pinpoint one aspect of my life leading to where I am now, it would probably be track. Trust me I would LOVE to run for you. I would love to run at Heps, at Penn Relays. I would love to run a 4:40 mile. That was my goal coming into college. But everything seemed to be thrown at me so quickly that I feel like I've dug myself so deep and at this point, right now there isn't any coming back. While I feel as if leaving the team would be a huge disappointment to you, my high school coach, my parents, my team and maybe even to myself, I've thought long and hard about this and feel that I just need to take the semester off to figure out what I really want in life and who I really am. As I said sports have always defined me, but here it hasn't brought me happiness. And it's time to define myself. All I need is a new beginning here and I think this semester will give me a chance to start over.

"Coach Martin gave me a book to read over break and it made me want to run even less, but I read some of it. One part particularly stuck out to me:

On the third day his outlook would begin to darken. For one thing, he was getting very, very tired. No particular day wore him out, but the accumulation of steady mileage began to take its toll. He never quite recovered fully between workouts and soon found himself walking around in a more-or-less constant state of fatigue-depression, a phase Denton called 'breaking down.' The new runner would find it more tedious than he could bear . . . at that point most of them would drift away. They would search within themselves somewhere along a dusty ten-mile trail or during the bad part of a really gut-churning 440 on the track, and find some key element missing. Sheepishly they would begin to miss workouts, then stop showing up altogether. They would convince themselves: there must be another way, there HAS to be. The attrition rate was nearly 100 percent.

"I hope you understand. I'm sorry to put you in this position and I don't expect you to be pleased to hear this, but the only thing I really want is a break. Maybe taking this semester off will make me realize I want to be on the team again and compete next year, but as of right now I strongly believe that isn't the right choice for me."

Maddy exhaled. She had said it—all of it. She put away the letter.

Often, quitting is a mistake. So much is learned through perseverance. Nearly every college coach has been in this situation: sitting across from a student-athlete who no longer wants to compete. Occasionally this is precisely what that young person needs. But more often, if student-athletes push through the discomfort of the first year, they grow stronger, and later, those thoughts of quitting come to seem like the notions of someone else entirely. They end up being thankful to the coach who saw a different path, one that kept them steadily directed toward their goals. How does a coach know which athletes to let walk away and which ones to fight for? They don't; they can't. Not for sure, anyway. They just do their best. "As a coach and a person who works with young people, the most important work we do is supporting people during that transition and to help them adjust to a new place, a new team, new academics," Dolan said. "It's always been important to me."

That morning inside the conference room, Dolan offered Maddy a different path, one that Stacy assumed her daughter couldn't see, or hadn't considered. Maybe her future on the team didn't have to be black or white. Perhaps they could take it slowly and she could call the shots, deciding over the next few weeks when and how she wanted to train. He had heard her: she needed a break, absolutely. But perhaps they could build that break into the larger structure of track, so she didn't have to quit entirely. In an effort to empower Maddy and restore her ownership of her athletic future, he turned over all decision making to her. "He said, 'If you're not happy with Coach Martin training you, I'll train you,'" said Stacy. "'If you're unhappy where you're living, I'll help you move.' He said she could stay on the track team and just train and not compete, or she could even pick the events she wanted to run. He was just so sweet and accommodating." But Maddy may not have felt empowered; she may only have felt the walls of the cage taking a new shape around her.

After offering all these new options, Coach Dolan placed

the decision in Maddy's hands. Stacy, too, thought these new options might help soothe Maddy without stripping her of her athletic identity. Dolan even offered an additional olive branch: taking it easy for the next few days, and then meeting again at the end of the week. Added Stacy: "He said, 'If you want to quit track, that's your decision, but obviously I would love for you to stay.'"

The two adults looked at Maddy.

Was there another choice? Was there a way to form the words "I can't keep running" and then, even harder, make those words come out of her mouth? She couldn't imagine it, so she said the only thing she could picture herself saying: "Okay, I'll try."

They say quitting is easy, and sometimes it is. Other times it's not. Other times it's the hardest thing of all—impossible, really. "You see someone young and talented and successful as Maddy was, and you care for her, and you're seeing this bright future," Dolan recalled. "And you can't fathom that she felt differently about things than anything we can see."

Because still, there on the horizon, looms another truth: depression and anxiety are not cured in a moment, with a single decision, though sometimes it can feel as if they might be. Even if Maddy had followed through on her decision to quit, other hard decisions would have followed. No matter how assiduously she had laid the groundwork for leaving, she hadn't yet experienced what that would be like.

★ ★ ★

On the way out of the office, Maddy took the letter, tore the two pages in half, and dropped them in a wastebasket. Mackenzie saw her mom and sister appear, and stood up. "What happened?" she asked.

"Wow, he is one fabulous coach," her mom was saying to Maddy as Mackenzie joined them. "Not many coaches would be like that, especially after how hard he recruited you."

"Are you still on the team?" Mack asked.

"Yup," Maddy said.

"Wait, you are? But...can I read the letter?" Mack asked.

"I already threw it out," replied Maddy.

The three of them walked over to the quad, where they met Ingrid, then went to her dorm room. "What happened?" Ingrid asked. "Did you quit?" They had planned to quit together, Maddy and Ingrid, both of them convinced that more free time would make them happier. Problem was, only Ingrid had followed through; only Ingrid had actually quit.

Maddy recounted the meeting. Dolan had offered her the world. And she couldn't disappoint him, you know? Plus, he had solved so many of her problems. She could make this new arrangement work; it was the best of both worlds. "I would say Madison seemed a little less troubled than before and during the meeting," Stacy remembered. "Almost like she felt better after expressing her feelings to us. However, looking back on it, I recall something felt amiss: when I said goodbye to her that day, I hugged her and of course I cried. I can't remember if she cried also, but in retrospect, her relief did seem short-lived."

A never-ending struggle: watching your child fumbling, forging a path, becoming an adult, and not being sure when they need you to hug them and keep them safe, and when they need you to let them be.

Once Stacy and Mackenzie had left, Maddy and Ingrid went over to a friend's dorm room.

1/13/14 8:13 PM

Maddy: Drinking w girls in Annabelle's room

Mack: No parties?

Maddy: Nopeeeee

Mack: Why

Maddy: Not a lot of people back on campus

Maddy: Mack I don't wanna do track at all anymore

Maddy: Seriously

Mack: Why?

Maddy: I hate it

The following morning, Maddy sent a message to a Penn friend who was on the football team, as well as to Trisha, a good friend from home. The day after that, she received an e-mail from Dolan laying out the plan for the upcoming week of training. So what, exactly, had changed?

1/14/14 10:04 AM

Maddy: Heading back today!?!

Logan: About to land ☺ 🔫

Logan: How'd meeting your coach go?

Maddy: Ehhh. As of now I'm still on the team but I'm meeting with him again on Thursday. I feel bad because he is soooo nice and so awesome and genuine and pretty much one of the reasons why I came to Penn in the first place so I feel really bad disappointing him. But I just don't enjoy training anymore. Like IDDDDDDKKKKKK I hate this so much

Logan: Did you say you wanted to leave the team? How are you still on it? Lol

Maddy: Yeah I did!! I legit wrote a two page letter about it. 2 pages!! But I'll explain the whole thing in a little when I get to the nail salon hahah

Maddy: Hi. Okk so pretty much told him my feelings about everything and was 100 percent honest about how I was feeling and he basically like felt guilty but also felt like I should have told him how I was feeling earlier. But he said that he would love to be my main coach so he just wants me to give it a shot for the rest of the semester instead of taking the semester off as like a break. So I'm meeting with him on Thursday again. But

I went to practice yesterday and really just didn't enjoy it. Like I don't think things are gonna change. I just don't know how to express that to him without feeling guilty or like a disappointment to him.

1/14/14 11:38 PM

Trisha: U looked like you were having fun in yo Snapchat

Maddy: Yeah I went to da bars 😊 but I'm still on the fence about track. The meeting went so well but like my coach (the head coach) is so friggin nice and awesome and a genuinely good person and I feel like it'd be a huge disappointment to him if I quit. I know I have to make this decision for me and do what's best to make me happy here but I just honestly feel like I'd be letting him down. And my parents.

Maddy: But I really don't enjoy it anymore

Trisha: Yeah I get what you mean but like you said you can't be unhappy just so you don't temporarily disappoint other people. Your parents will get over it I promise and the coach goes through stuff like that all the time he literally signed up for it when he became a coach. It's your life you need to do what makes ya happy ya feel

On Jan 15, 2014, at 1:00 PM, "Stephen Dolan" wrote:

All,

We have the Air Structure reserved today from 3:30 to 5:00. Let's plan to meet there at 3:15 for practice. The plan is to take a distance run locally and meet back at the Air Structure at 4:30 for an organized team strength training circuit.

Here is the general plan for the next few days:

Thursday: Van out from Dunning at 3:15

Friday: Meet at Air Structure at 3:15 to warm-up for the workout (Weather permitting we will run the workout on the outdoor track) (5-6 x 1000 at 5K pace w/ 2:00 rest)

Saturday: OYO for cross training or a recovery run and some core work

Sunday: Van out to the park at 10:00 AM

Goal setting for 2014

Also, as I mentioned in our full team meeting on Monday, I feel that it is very important to set some concrete goals as we embark on the track season. I'd like each of you to take a few minutes to write down 2-3 specific competitive goals that you have for this year on the track. At least one or two of these goals should be a specific time that you are dreaming about running. I'd also like to see you brainstorm in regard to what are the key things that you need to do to achieve your goal. For Example: "I want to break a 5:00 mile and I see my sleep schedule and better consistency with my strength training as important areas in which I can improve to help me chase this goal."

You don't have to share your goals with me but I would love to hear one or two of them if you are willing to share so I have a better understanding of what you are dreaming about. Please send me a short goals e-mail if you would like to share. I'd love to help you achieve your goals and want to have fun in the pursuit.

Proposed Haverford Meet Entry

Men's 3000: VA, WM, CN, Bsh, JT, NT, LW

Men's Mile: TA, ED, CP, TS, CSh, BSm

Women's 3000: KJ, Cleo, Clarissa

Women's Mile: SMc, EG, AM

TBD: MD, AD, EQ, **MH**, NG

Dreamscapes

It is the middle of the night. I am suddenly awake. Or have I been awake for a while but it was so dark I believed I was asleep? I don't know where I am. But I'm not concerned.

I reach for my computer. I don't usually do that. But there is something on there I need, though I'm not sure what. I pull my silver Mac from the bedside table and onto the sheets. The room is ink black. I open the laptop, and a halo of light appears.

The artificial glow is jarring. I rub my eyes. I blink.

What am I looking for?

I scan the icons on the desktop. None are what I want. I look at the dashboard, scroll through the applications. I carefully consider each. I'm definitely looking for something. My mouse scrolls over Reminders, then Notes, then FaceTime.

I pause. FaceTime. Is that what I want?

I launch the application. The icon bounces on the dashboard. It seems like it might not start. I bring my mouse to the top left corner of the screen so I can quit the launch. I am impatient. If this isn't what I'm looking for, something else is. I must find it.

Just before I scroll down to Quit FaceTime, the app opens. I almost quit anyway. But I don't. The green light goes on above my camera. A black box appears on my screen. I expect to see myself.

But I don't.

I see Maddy.

She is wearing a Penn track jacket. Her hair is pulled back. She is smiling and talking to someone, but I don't have audio. Why am I getting her FaceTime feed? It is as if we are screen mirroring, or as if someone—Was it me? Did I do this?—hacked her computer, rerouted everything to mine.

I consider ending the call. But I do not. I am mesmerized. She is so bright and full of life. She is in a hotel room. She is sitting on the bed. The headboard is behind her, a piece of bad art above. I try turning up the volume, but it is already on max. Maddy is telling a story. She gestures a lot. Then she laughs. I know that it is a good sound even though I cannot hear it.

What magic has brought this to me? I don't care. I don't move. I don't want a single molecule disturbed.

Maddy listens to whoever is on the other line. She speaks occasionally. She nods. After a minute, the conversation starts winding down. I can tell. And it makes me sad. Maddy is leaning forward. She smiles, waves.

Then she hits the end button.

I realize I have been bracing for her disappearance. But she doesn't disappear. I don't understand, but I know instantly that Maddy is unaware the camera is still on. She has ended the call. The camera should be off. But it is not.

I lean forward.

She inhales deeply. As she exhales, the brightness leaks from her face. Her elbow is on her knee. She raises her hand to her forehead. I can't see her eyes. A minute later, her shoulders begin to shake. She wipes tears from her eyes. She is staring just off camera, at something much farther away than could be possible.

My heart begins thudding. I play with the settings. I turn on my microphone. I call her name. I touch the screen.

She still cannot hear me.

Tears keep falling from her eyes. So many that she stops trying to wipe them away. She seems to have forgotten she is crying. It's like she's not even there, not really.

I thought I was getting closer to her. I thought I was closer than I had ever been. I could finally see her. She was right there, right there on my screen. Wasn't this intimacy?

But then it struck me as I quickly closed my computer:

She had never been farther away.

CHAPTER 9

The Picture

If one only wished to be happy, this could be easily accomplished; but we wish to be happier than other people, and this is always difficult, for we believe others to be happier than they are.

— *Montesquieu*

Lorraine Sullivan followed the social media feeds of her own kids as well as those of their friends. All the parents did. Free access, and thus free insight, into the thoughts and actions of the young people around them: what a gift and a reassurance, to be able to flip open her iPad or iPhone and know where the person she loved was, to know they were safe for at least another day.

The night of January 17, 2014, Emma Sullivan had just returned to Boston College for her second semester. Back in Allendale, Lorraine scrolled through feeds on her iPad and was stopped cold by the newest image posted by Maddy. She stared at the picture, absorbed it, allowed the energy of it to radiate through the screen. Exactly what was Maddy trying to say? A minute later, Lorraine returned to scrolling, but the aftertaste remained: *That photo is eerie.* The image made Maddy seem nostalgic for a time and place she had never seen. And if this was true, if she was, how would she ever stifle that longing?

This wasn't the first time an outsider, a parent, had felt that way about Maddy's social feed. Hers were more cryptic than the posts of other kids, more dependent on quotes, and views from high places; the images conveyed the feeling that Maddy was trying to say something, without knowing exactly how or what it was. What drifted from the screen was a kind of yearning, a wandering energy—something crucial had been lost, but not quite found.

A searching energy permeates almost every young person's social media. After all, what is a social feed if not a journal, but in digital, visual form? Perhaps the most important distinguishing feature of a social account is its public nature, the understanding each user has, from the moment of launch, that everything is for public consumption. But perhaps we are overstating the effect of this distinction: If in private, most of us allow ourselves to say or write certain truths we otherwise wouldn't, then perhaps the reverse holds true. Perhaps we share things in public that we couldn't offer in private. If we've accepted that we are different in private, is this not also true for how we reveal ourselves in public? And which version of ourselves is more real?

As young people, we are trying to find our voice: trying out who we are, again and again, until something feels more accurate than the previous thing. Yet we rarely admit—or even recognize—that this is what we're doing. On social media, few people confess that they've poured immense time and energy into what they post. We don't confess this because we assume we're the only ones who fret over such trivial things. Because nobody could possibly be as self-conscious as we are. We believe what we see. And we can't be what we can't see. We are so credulous when we assume that everyone else must be the version of themselves they portray in public, even if we are hardly the people we present ourselves as.

We put time into our social media because we believe that it affords us the unique opportunity to fashion our own identity. We care about the images we post and the lines we write underneath those images, because it's all part of reflecting who we are and constructing who we want to become. Would you put more time, or less, into a post if you knew it was your last? Would you want the image and words to be perfect, an ideal lasting representation of you, or would you quickly recognize the futility of the pursuit, that the whole thing was a mirage merely reflecting distorted images of the real world? And would you instead spend your time absorbing the world itself?

On the night of January 17, Maddy took a series of photos of Rittenhouse Square, in downtown Philadelphia, on her iPhone. She was standing on the dead grass behind the main walkways in the park, behind the benches on which people lounge during spring and summer, and huddle during winter. Lights are dangling from the sparse trees, the beauty of the holiday season still radiating at dusk. The first photo Maddy took is cloudy in the lens, exuding dreariness. Her second photo showed nearly the exact same scene. In that image, an older couple is walking through the frame: the woman is wearing a red coat, the man a green coat and hat. The couple is in motion, a soft blur coming off each of them. In the final photo Maddy took, the couple is gone.

It is this last photo that Maddy began editing. She made the colors pop; the benches go from dull brown to a fiery red; the lights morph from small pops to glowing, gorgeous lanterns. And the night behind the foreground went from looking just like any other to appearing as something spectacular—a city park placed underwater, submerged, radiating.

This was not a picture of the real world, but a picture of what Maddy wished the real world looked like. "I tell my kids all the time: You have to decide how you're going to filter the world," Lorraine says. "You have to check yourself

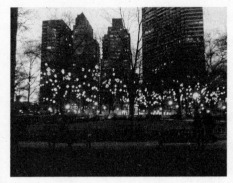
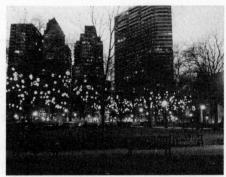

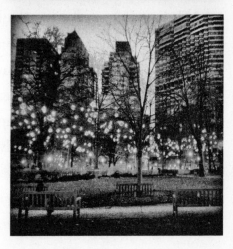

Three versions of Rittenhouse Square, as shot and edited by Maddy on January 17; the picture on the right appeared on her Instagram account. *(Madison Holleran)*

daily—what am I making of everything I'm seeing? Does everything they're seeing have to be as good as everything we expect of them? I think we tell our kids they have to be really, really good at all these things. I think it's rampant, especially in these affluent suburbs. This generation, everybody is supposed to be good at everything. But God forbid if you're not. I tell my kids: I went to college. Nobody took us on college tours. They were just like, 'You want to go to college?' And they would drop you off and that was it. Nobody checked in on everybody, all day every day. The difference is astounding. Everybody is hovering over these kids. Are you winning at every game? Are exams going well? What are you doing with your free time? The pendulum has swung so far to the other side. I think it's backfiring."

On Wednesday night, January 15, Maddy went to a party with Ingrid. She was wearing black tights, a sweater, her black Nike running sneakers, and a black jacket. As the two friends were leaving the party in the small hours of Thursday morning, Ingrid took a photo of her friend. Madison is standing on the sidewalk, her right hand on her hip. Her mouth is smiling, but the photo isn't clear, and it's impossible to see if her eyes are, too.

While at the party, Maddy had taken a few photos, most with Ingrid. She picked her favorite, one of just the two of them, a young man grinning in the background. Maddy filtered the image, popping the colors, then texted it to her friend Justine.

Maddy: Do u like this enough to Insta?

Everything is filtered, either on the way in or on the way out, or in both directions. This includes practically everything Maddy did: the interaction when sitting in front of the therapist, or in Emma's kitchen with her best friend. But at least in those, Maddy could not hide so easily behind a second digital filter. She could not hide behind the breezy lightness of an added emoji: a monkey covering its eyes, or an "lol" or "hahahaha," which she casually added to almost all her texts.

Is there a human, in-person equivalent of a monkey covering its eyes? If someone says to you, in person, that they hate where they are, or what they're doing, or what their life has become, could they make those words softer with any kind of specific facial expression? Would it even matter if they tried? You would still be in front of them, reading their energy and emotion, and the smile on their lips would be false, incapable of dispelling their desperate energy.

We have translated expressions and emotions into emojis, and simply using an emoji seems to tell the recipient that all is okay. The inclusion of even one of those animated faces signals ease and lightness, regardless of what emotion the emoji represents, even if it represents crying. The acronym LOL rarely means laughing out loud—not literally laughing out loud, anyway. Very little of what we say in text is a literal representation of how we feel, what we're doing, how we're behaving. It's an animated, easy-to-digest version: an exaggeration or a simplification, but not a reflection. And that would be fine if it weren't the main way we now communicate with one another. We believe we're communicating with the humans we love and adore, and we are. But we aren't absorbing their humanity.

Emoji is the world's first digital universal language, and

it's frighteningly superficial. Ironically, emojis are devoid of real emotion. Maddy was in constant contact with dozens of friends and family, a skimming of the surface covering miles and miles of ground but very little depth. And through all those messages to all those people, thousands and thousands of communications, almost nobody noticed anything significantly amiss.

Before returning to Penn in January, Maddy asked her parents if she could take with her a picture of herself as a kid, holding a tennis racquet. She asked for duct tape, which went unused. And eventually, at some point before she left her dorm room on January 17, she opened her MacBook and wiped her Internet history. She was preparing for what had been simmering on the back burner; she was moving it to the front.

Anticipation

Anticipation is one of the best parts of life. When I was twenty-two years old, I quit my job playing professional basketball in Ireland, but before I retreated home to the States, head down, embarrassed, I disappeared on a backpacking trip through Europe. I took a cheap flight from Dublin to Paris, then a train to Milan, then one to Rome, Rome being in my mind the climax of this spontaneous journey. I had studied Latin for three years. And after that, or perhaps because of that, I became fascinated with the Roman Empire, in particular the Colosseum. I kept a journal on this trip, and I remember pulling out that small black notebook while sitting in my seat on the train, watching the Italian countryside pass. I wrote, detailing on those pages how I assumed the Colosseum would make me feel. I had conjured images of it, an approximation, from all the movies and news stories and pictures in textbooks I had seen over the years. And I explained to myself, writing sentence after sentence, what it would feel like to stand inside a piece of history: I imagined the collective energy of the millions who had come before, who had passed through the same space. I imagined that this energy, like a ghost, would make my hair stand on end. I would hear the echoes of those ancient crowds, bloodthirsty, human, wanting. I imagined myself standing within this swirl of energy and emotion, as this was a place that had housed so much of both.

I never imagined feeling nothing. And yet, once the train pulled into Rome and I wended my way to the Colosseum, I remember standing inside, and there it was, an emotion impossible not to name: disappointment. The birds chirped. The sky was a lovely blue with the occasional milky cloud. Beads of sweat pinned my shirt to my back. I looked around at the crumbling structure, at the other people exploring the space. I closed my eyes. I willed something, anything, to wash over me. Nothing did. I was still just—me. The same me, with the same worries and concerns and hopes, the ones that somehow I had imagined would be made small by the force of history. My anxiety over quitting basketball in Ireland, and how puzzling my future now appeared to me, had dislodged me from the present. I felt very much like an astronaut slowly floating away from her spaceship, desperate for a force to push me back to safety. Somehow I had hoped that standing in the Colosseum would be like consulting a medium, allowing me to stand among the collective yearning of the masses. And this would make me feel less alone, would be the gust that pushed me back to safety. But I was unchanged. After a while I left the famous structure, and on my walk to the hostel where I was staying, I bought an apple from a corner store. It tasted the same as any other.

On the train back to Paris, I again pulled out my notebook and attempted to explain what I had felt, and what I had not felt, and why I had not felt it, and what that lack of feeling might mean. And I landed on one specific thing: perhaps some things really are better left to the imagination.

When I got home to the States, one of my friends asked about my backpacking trip. I explained the highlights and the adventure, and then I said, "But I went to the Colosseum and, I don't know, it just didn't do anything for me. I had built it up in my mind I guess, but I just stood there, disappointed." My friend looked at me and frowned, and in that second I considered for the first time that maybe blame for the disappointment I had felt lay not with the Colosseum, but with me. My friend then said, "I've always wanted to go to Rome—don't bum me out!"

From then on, when people asked about my trip and I showed them pictures—the tangible kind, from those yellow disposable cameras—if they asked how amazing the Colosseum was, I found myself lying, saying, "Amazing—so amazing." I had somehow decided it was my social and moral obligation to have loved this trip, loved this adventure, and specifically loved the Colosseum, so as not to rob others of even a moment of that vicarious, transferrable excitement—of their own joy of anticipation. And also, expressing any kind of disappointment with a trip to Rome is unpopular, especially when articulated to anyone who hasn't been lucky enough to go.

I tell this story to illustrate that all of us feel an obligation to optimism and happiness when we're around others. If you break down my trip to the Colosseum, which occurred before the advent of social media and smartphones, you'll notice that my behavior—before, during, and after—almost mimics the way I would act today. As I approached the structure, I built it up in my mind by writing it into life to pique my own interest. Today, I'd likely look through tagged pictures of the location on Instagram. After my visit, I quickly shifted to telling a superficial but upbeat story about the moment, not very different from what I might do now, which is tag myself on Instagram in a picture at the landmark with the hashtag "amazing."

The main, glaring difference between now and then is that in 2005, I was at least somewhat present during the moment I was actually standing in the Colosseum. I took one or two pictures on my camera, but I wasn't considering the social capital of an Instagram post from that geo-tagged location. I had enough space to consider myself in relation to the millions of ancient Romans who had climbed those steps (even if I failed in fully connecting to that history). Now, today, I fear I would only consider all the others who were Instagramming from there and elsewhere, and how the image I produced might compare. Eventually, the story of my 2005 trip to the Colosseum would become a kind of performance—but it wasn't yet, not while I stood inside those ancient ruins, feeling not much of anything.

The best part of life is often the way we anticipate what is to come. For a trip, for the weekend, for a party, for so many moments that are happening after and apart from the ones we are currently living. Sometimes we also believe that another place will change us, or at least how we feel, and that it will be a change for the better. And even if we recognize, when we get to this time or place, that it has not changed us, that we are still just ourselves, we cannot help but fall for this trick the next time, and again and again afterward. We fall for it because it soothes us during all the moments we aren't doing exactly the thing we wish we could be doing, and because it allows us the transcendent emotion of anticipation. Anticipation allows us to be in two different moments at once. But it is often a zero-sum game: we steal from one to fuel the other.

In the poem "Questions of Travel" by Elizabeth Bishop, she writes the following: "Is it right to be watching strangers in a play / in this strangest of theatres? / What childishness is it that while there's a breath of life / in our bodies, we are determined to rush / to see the sun the other way around?"

Anticipation fuels optimism, at least temporarily. We tell ourselves that the current moment will not last forever, that the next moment will deliver us somewhere better. Of course, if that promise is repeatedly broken, if those next moments are never better, a kind of melancholy can set in: both our present and future seem tarnished.

Isn't social media fueled by anticipation? A world exists in our phone, which we can retreat to—an escape that might offer us something more pleasant, or at least a distraction from our momentary boredom at being a human who is alive in the world, and therefore dealing with all the things that come with that. Social media reflects our actual existence, but feels freer: not mired in tangible weight and sweat and fear and sadness. Social media is a picture of the Colosseum in glorious lighting, with an upbeat hashtag; it's not the friend standing in front of you, dismayed at her inexplicable disappointment.

In the fall of 2015, I guest-taught a freshman class at Columbia University. Approximately twenty-five students had read "Split Image" as well as a collection of essays by Susan Sontag, *On Photography*. The idea was to introduce to the students the concept that photographs, though seemingly unbiased, are often manipulated as much as, if not more than, words. Sontag writes:

Even when photographers are most concerned with mirroring reality, they are still haunted by tacit imperatives of taste and conscience. The immensely gifted members of the Farm Security Administration photographic project of the late 1930s (among them Walker Evans, Dorothea Lange, Ben Shahn, Russell Lane) would take dozens of frontal pictures of one of their sharecropper subjects until satisfied that they had gotten just the right look on film—the precise expression on the subject's face that supported their own notions about poverty, light, dignity, texture, exploitation, and geometry. In deciding how a picture should look, in preferring one exposure to another, photographers are always imposing standards on their subjects. Although there is a sense in which the camera does indeed capture reality, not just interpret it, photographs are as much an interpretation of the world as paintings and drawings are.

One key word exists in the above Sontag quote: *conscience*. During our conversation at Columbia, the students mined how they felt about social media, and they kept striking on a similar concept: obligation. So many of these college freshmen felt a moral obligation to project a certain kind of happiness. They could not, as one student put it, "in good conscience" disseminate sadness and unhappiness into the world. Because they chose to remain conscious, they participated in a performance meant to make the collective comfortable, but which came at personal cost—a cost often small, but occasionally great. The layers of ethical issues are numerous. Some of us could be sharing "just to do it," but the fact of our sharing will evoke in others feelings and ideas about the way the world works. Our posts are part of an ecosystem: we are all engaged in creating a story that reacts to the stories around us. Then if you dig one layer deeper, we are dealing with another variable. Before we share, we engage in a conversation with ourselves about what kind of image of ourselves we are placing in the world and what the image must mean to us as it relates to the world. Social media is a form of offense and defense: we consume, we absorb, and we decide what to consume and absorb based on what we've consumed and absorbed.

Inside that small Columbia classroom, we started discussing this cycle at a granular level. We experience a moment emotionally. And during many such moments, we often consciously capture an image, the content of which is often the most appealing interpretation of the moment. Then we make an intellectual choice about if, and how, to share that image, a decision often but not always influenced by the moral obligation we feel to contribute positively to society. After we share the image, we monitor the feedback on the post, which will influence our understanding of what does and doesn't resonate, and what we might share next time. Then the cycle starts again. We start viewing our world through the lens of what shares well—a hybrid reality in which people and locations and pops of color exist both in our tangible world and also as backgrounds for images that will share well. In other words, when you walk through Central Park, you are partially absorbing the sights and sounds of being alive, and you are also pasting items, in your mind's eye, into a potential social post. Perhaps we are now all like walking versions of those collages we used to make—the ones that incorporated real photographs as well as idealized magazine cutouts and headlines.

The question bouncing around the minds of these students was more about effect than about process: Were they emotionally experiencing life differently because of this cycle? Was it eroding the quality of their experiences? When you are not concerned with sharing every moment with hundreds (or thousands, or millions) of others, does the moment belong to you in a more profound way? Sometimes when we talk of Hollywood stars, we hypothesize that all of the pictures they've had taken of themselves, those posed for and those stolen, have somehow zapped them of an unquantifiable essence, like a distant cousin of what happens to the photographs themselves, which fade over time. If you share a picture of yourself eating pie, instead of simply enjoying the pie in real time, is your absorption of the sensation diluted?

A few hours after the class at Columbia, I was walking along the Gowanus Canal, in Brooklyn, talking to my dad. The sun was bright in the sky, and I remember looking at the light reflecting off the usually dense, murky canal water, and I remember considering for the first time that this dingy body of water was actually appealing in its own, flawed way. (Ever since that day, I've looked at the Gowanus differently—seen it as a kind of artwork, a literal absorption of the city it runs through.)

As I was watching light bounce off the canal, I was telling my dad about the class, and about Maddy and what she must have been feeling and thinking. He had listened to me on this topic many times over the months, but on this day, after I stopped talking, he didn't reply. I waited for one beat, then another. I flexed my foot on the bottom rung of the railing that kept me from tumbling into the water.

"You there?" I finally asked.

"Yeah, I'm here," he said, then paused again. "Just do me a favor, okay? Take care of yourself. Promise me that if you start feeling down, you'll tell me."

"Oh, Dad," I said. "I'm okay; I promise."

"But—do you see yourself in Madison? Is that it?"

"I mean, I guess in some ways, yes," I said. "In some ways, I think I know exactly what she was going through, because I've been through the same thing. But then when it comes to how she seems to have interpreted these things, how they *felt* to her—well, that's where I stop seeing myself in Maddy."

The response I gave my dad that afternoon is almost

entirely accurate. Of course, if I mine deeper, I can find a connecting thread that helps me fully understand, even if tuning in to the frequency of that connection feels fleeting and distant, nearly abstract.

Crushing, debilitating anxiety has descended on me only once. I have battled everyday anxiety on occasions too numerous to count, whether before speaking in public, before going on TV, before offering an opinion in meetings. Yet during each of these occasions I understood, even as the weight of the fear commandeered a good portion of my brain and body, that the panic was temporary, circumstantial. The anxiety had a shelf life; of this I was sure.

But on one specific winter morning—the catalyst was the implosion of a relationship the night before—I awoke before dawn and, as I came to consciousness, experienced a blend of frenzied thinking and an overwhelming physical malaise that catapulted me into a state of panic. I tried breathing deeply, but my mind continued churning: *What's the point of all this? Who am I now? What does my future hold? Am I alone in the world? Will I always be alone? Aren't we all, essentially, alone?* I actually started talking aloud to myself, telling myself to calm down, that it would pass. But this self-talk failed. My heart continued racing, even though I hadn't gotten out of bed yet—had barely even moved. I reached for an empty journal I keep on my nightstand; I tried to write my way out of the moment, believing that perhaps I could exorcise the thoughts, silence them by dragging them from my head to the paper, where they would wither and die in the open air. After writing furiously for seven pages, my handwriting slanted and messy, the ink blotting, I closed the journal and waited. I shut my eyes. The panic was still there. *Is this feeling real?* I asked myself. *And do I have any control over it?* It seemed as if I should have more control, for who could control it, who could make it go away, if not me?

I tried allowing the panic to just wash over me. Perhaps, I told myself, resisting the emotions was a mistake. *Just feel it all,* I told myself, *then you'll be done with it.* For an hour I lay on my back, blankly staring at the white ceiling. At one point I curled up into a ball, hoping that anxiety was like nausea, and that mimicking life in the womb would ease the symptoms. Eventually I remember screaming into my hands, actually saying aloud, "What the fuck!"

The sun came up, and the city outside my window started making its usual noises: the F train running along the tracks, engines starting, the distant blaring of horns along the Brooklyn-Queens Expressway. I remember, prone in my bed, looking at these noises—or, rather, looking at the drawn off-white shade, behind which was the window, behind which was the world from which these noises were emanating. I usually love these sounds: they're proof of ordered chaos, of life and hope and optimism. But that morning the noises struck me as random and pointless, and if I'd had the power, I would have silenced all of it. The dull yellow of the early morning sun had backlit the drawn shade, and the whole image, which I'd seen and appreciated a hundred mornings before, disgusted me. Not a minute later, as I lay on my side, my pillow tucked under my ear, a thought came screaming around the corner of my mind and ran me over before I could dodge it: *Holy shit, I can't live like this.* "This" had been going on for only three hours, and it was scaring me; *I* was scaring me.

I called my mom. I started crying. She took the next train from Albany down to the city. She hugged me when I collected her at Penn Station. We walked to get coffee. I tried to explain what I was feeling, what had happened. Nothing, not even the comfort of my mom, could calm me. That night, hours later, we decided to go see a movie, and at some point in the darkness of the theater, I could feel the fear start to seep out of my body. I tried not to pay it much mind in case my attention might halt the flow, but by movie's end I had returned to a state of equilibrium that I vowed never again to take for granted. And to this day, when I see the poster for the movie we went to see that night, a mix of emotions bubble up, but the dominant one is gratitude that this bout of panic lasted only twelve hours. (Over the next few weeks I had random bursts of anxiety, but never again did it seem to coil around my heart the way it did that first morning.)

I do not live with daily, steady anxiety and depression; therefore I cannot know what life feels like if you do. But I know this: Madison walked a path. And at first, the path she walked is familiar to me: the sun is high; the grass is matted; the underbrush is tame. I've walked that path, or something similar. Then, at some point, the conditions start to change; they become more ominous, denser, less traveled. Then, farther ahead, the path appears to shape-shift—it's not subject to the same laws of physics, of life. I can peer ahead into the distance and see the outline of where Maddy walked, but I cannot report back from the inside. For most of us, understanding how much of this path we've traveled is impossible: it's a road of unknown length.

CHAPTER 10

Spruce and 15th

The Lehigh women's soccer coach, Eric Lambinus, was sitting outside Fado, an Irish pub in downtown Philadelphia, talking on the phone with his wife, when he spotted a familiar face walking toward him and quickly told his wife he would need to call her back. In town for a coaching convention, he and his assistant coach, Amy Huff, were at Fado with Mike Bend, who at the time coached the school's men's soccer team. "Maddy!" Eric called, right after hanging up with his wife. He began walking across the street toward her.

The coach couldn't help but feel that spotting Maddy was a stroke of good fortune: perhaps their crossing paths was serendipitous. He and the rest of Lehigh's coaching staff had been disappointed when she'd changed her mind at the end of the recruiting process, backing out of her verbal commitment and deciding to run track instead of play soccer.

They believed she would have been a very good college player.

Eric had also heard through the grapevine—players on his team still kept in touch with Maddy, as well as with Maddy's friends—that she wasn't happy at Penn. Neither Eric nor Amy had any additional details about her situation, including whether she might legitimately consider transferring or if her malaise simply represented the usual freshman ups and downs. Maybe if she did want to leave, they had a chance—a second chance. They also wanted to know how she was doing, as both Eric and Amy had spent hours on the phone with her, had gotten to know her well—better than most recruits—and were genuinely interested in whether she was enjoying her first year of college. They both liked her.

Madison lifted her head upon hearing her name. She spotted Eric, the coach she had almost gone to play for out of high school. He was crossing the street toward her. In her right hand, she was holding a shopping bag.

For much of the afternoon, Maddy had responded to her phone messages, but at some point she had stopped looking at the new texts as they popped up. Earlier that day, after finishing class, she had begun rewriting the script for her Friday afternoon and evening. None of these changes seemed premeditated or planned in advance, but as she began rearranging things, she couldn't bring herself to casually text, to continue seeing the names of her friends and family. She had made the decision to separate herself from them, and that separation started when she stopped responding on her phone.

The night before, she and Ingrid had watched the remake of *The Parent Trap*. The two friends had parted ways early, since Maddy had morning obligations: a test to take, as well as a lifting workout for the track team. When they had said goodbye, Ingrid had walked away believing she would see her friend the next night. The pair had continued texting the following afternoon, about which sororities they were most interested in. And as the afternoon wore on, Ingrid finally asked if she was definitely seeing Maddy that night. But to this final text, Maddy didn't respond.

Ingrid: Taylor and I have exactly the same except our first and second are swapped

Maddy at 12:14: Did not everyone get all six? Ahh mines diff. Whaaaat I wonder how that worked out

Ingrid at 3:52: Idkk are you done with class?

Maddy at 5:36: Ahh yes sorry I went running

Maddy: Whatcha doing

Ingrid at 6:17: Thoughts on going out
tonight?

Although Maddy told Ingrid she had gone running that afternoon, it's unclear if she actually had, because she also sent an e-mail to Steve Dolan in the middle of the afternoon, when she would have been running, asking if she could opt out of the afternoon workout.

On Jan. 17, 2014, at 2:07 PM, Madison wrote:

Hi! My legs are still pretty sore so could I just do the bike again today and then do a workout tomorrow?

From: Stephen Dolan
Date: Fri, Jan. 17, 2014 at 3:29 PM

Madison,

Ok. Let's talk on the phone later about the plan for this weekend.

Call me anytime after 7:00.

Coach

Madison never called Dolan. Ingrid believed she was meeting up with Maddy that night after each of them continued rush, which was set to begin at 6 p.m. at Houston Hall. Actually, Maddy should have been at Houston Hall right about the time she ran into Eric. She had received a reminder e-mail about the event less than two hours before.

Instead of being on campus at that moment, Maddy was on a downtown Philly street corner, watching Eric walk toward her. She hadn't expected to see anyone, let alone the soccer coach she had spurned in favor of Penn, but now there was no way to avoid him, since they'd made eye contact and he had called her name. She was wearing jeans and a sweater, a coat—just an everyday outfit, not athletic gear.

Eric and Maddy walked across the street to join Amy and Mike. After the standard greetings, Eric asked Maddy what she was doing alone downtown on a Friday night.

"Just doing some shopping," Maddy told him, lifting the bag in her hand.

"Get anything good?" he asked.

"Just some gifts for my family," she said.

She had actually bought the gifts earlier in the day, at the U of Penn Bookstore. While she was there her dad had called, which was not unusual: everyone was worried about her and checking in several times a day. Jim wanted to know if she'd made any progress on finding a therapist in Philly. Both Jim and Stacy had agreed that, along with the counselor she was seeing at home, Maddy needed professional help from someone near school.

Madison told her dad that she hadn't yet found a therapist

in Philly, but that she would. And maybe she planned to find one, in the same way she was still planning for second semester, still rushing sororities and inquiring about a room switch. Nothing is decided until it is. Yet she was at that very moment shopping for her family and friends. She bought Godiva chocolates for Jim. She bought a necklace for her mom. She bought gingersnaps for her grandparents, who always had that flavor in their home. She bought an outfit for Hayes, her nephew, who had been born two weeks earlier, on New Year's Eve. She had a copy of *The Happiness Project* for Ingrid, with a note scribbled inside. She also had that picture of herself as a young kid, holding a tennis racquet. She had shown that picture to her dad over holiday break and announced that she was borrowing it, that she needed it for something, though she didn't say for what. She also had a note she had written, trying to explain herself.

These were the items inside the shopping bag Maddy was holding as she spoke to Eric. Of course, Eric thought nothing of the exchange: he assumed the bag was filled with belated Christmas gifts.

"I heard things aren't going great at Penn," Eric said.

"Yeah, it's much different than I thought it would be," she said. "But I'm not sure what to do about it."

"Different how?" Eric asked.

"School is difficult, so much more than high school," Madison said. "All of it is really, really hard, plus I'm not enjoying track."

"Just have honest conversations with everyone about how things are going," he said. Then he added, "And if Penn isn't the school for you, that's okay—really. It will be okay."

Eric told her that options still existed, that just because she had chosen Penn first didn't mean she couldn't change her mind. A standard process existed if she wanted to transfer, and, yes, she needed to jump through the proper hoops, but that was always still an option. Eric wanted to be careful about what he was saying. He didn't want to be seen to be poaching a player from another school, but he also felt he knew Maddy, what drove her, and he had always believed she loved soccer. So he wanted to convey a simple message to her without saying the actual words: she could still come play soccer at Lehigh.

Maddy was noncommittal.

"How are you doing, though?" Eric asked again.

"Fine," she said, glancing at the server walking past. "I'm good."

"You sure?"

"Yeah," she looked down.

"Well, look, if you ever really need anything, please don't hesitate to call," Eric said. "You can always reach out."

"Thanks," Madison said, beginning to walk away. "I appreciate that."

"Good luck," Eric said.

"Good luck!" Amy echoed.

"Good seeing you," Madison said, then turned and continued down the street.

Once Madison was out of earshot, Eric and Amy explained to Mike the backstory: the aggressive recruitment, the verbal commitment, and the last-minute switch. Mike told the two coaches they had been nicer to Maddy than he might have been, given her behavior in the past, but the two coaches were too thrilled at the idea that they might have a second shot at Madison. "Amy and I both said we were really happy to see her," Eric later recalled. "We both kept talking about how great she would be for our team. She looked good; she looked fit. We were happy to see her, and it seemed like good fortune. We just thought it was meant to be, a little bit."

A few minutes later the three coaches went into Fado for dinner. When they left, about an hour and a half later, they noticed police cars blocking the street, but that was not unusual in Philadelphia. The group turned around and walked the long way, giving not another thought to the commotion.

The parking garage at the corner of Spruce and 15th is a block from Fado. The structure is nondescript: it's next to a Rita's, the famous Philly water ice chain, and the ground floor is occupied by a sports bar, Fox & Hound. In fact, the entire corner is unremarkable. There's a drugstore on one side, a dry cleaning joint down the street, and the Kimmel Center is adjacent—a lovely, looming building, but hardly magnificent. "We asked her Penn friends how she would know to go there, and they said they had no idea," Justine says. "It's not near Penn. I'm guessing she might have gone for a run or a walk one day. Or maybe she chose it that day. No one in Philly can make the connection."

One notable distinction exists. On the front of the parking garage is a small art installation. Painted onto the cement walls are fragments of phrases. The words conjure distinct images, and an energy emanates from the building that makes a passerby feel as if something within might be haunted. The artwork frames the entrance door to the parking garage, which leads to the interior stairs, which eventually lead to the top of the structure. The installation, called *Passing Through,* is one in a series of twenty throughout Philadelphia, the City of Murals.

The artwork on the parking garage consists of dozens of unconnected phrases, fleeting thoughts, stenciled onto the cement. One phrase, along the bottom of the wall, reads "She had wings on." Next to the words is a drawing of a woman with flowing hair who appears to be trapped in some metaphysical state, her eyes pressed closed, her hair unruly. At first glance the words on the building seem confusing: Do any relate? And if so, how?

The origin story of each *Passing Through* site starts with a tape recorder. A person standing at the site of the future artwork records the conversations of people as they pass. But because the person holding the recorder is stationary, only fragments of these conversations are caught, which produces a steady stream of seemingly unrelated words and thoughts.

On its website, *Passing Through* posted the text captured at each site. Here is a chunk of the conversations recorded at the parking garage at 15th and Spruce: "I try to live life as if tomorrow will never come good luck to you nice talking to you no one can compare cracks it open warm bottle the point is the other half wants to ask that question you know she constantly argues and fights I tell her all about the patient about an hour and 45 minutes later she doesn't answer my page could you give me all of them at once..."

Madison walked directly to this parking garage after running into Eric.

Before she left her dorm room that morning, she made her bed. She never made her bed. She also cleaned her side of the space and scribbled a note that she left in the room: "I don't know who I am anymore. Trying. Trying. Trying. I'm sorry. I love you... sorry again... sorry again... sorry again... How did this happen?"

Maddy had placed a second note inside the bag she was holding, tucked among the gifts for her family. She opened the door to the garage stairwell and climbed the nine flights to the top. Only one or two cars were parked on the top level because there were spots open below, so there was no need for drivers to circle all the way up. The pavement of the top level sloped upward toward the southern railing. The view of South Philly, of its twinkling lights, was arresting. Madison loved views. She loved images she could frame, that she could file away if only for a few moments in the cabinet of her mind. And the vista from this perch was vast; the tallest buildings were behind the viewer, so the twilight sky seemed to stretch all the way to Delaware. In a way, standing at the top of that parking garage felt like being inside a cube, but with one open side—the side Maddy was now facing. Every other direction consisted of tall buildings pressing against each other.

Madison placed the shopping bag on the ground. The note inside explained, as best she could, what was about to happen, but mostly the words provided a guide for something much less confusing: which gift was for whom.

She left the picture of herself as a kid with a tennis racquet tucked inside a copy of the young adult book *Reconstructing Amelia,* which tells the story of a devastated single mother who pieces together clues about the death of her daughter, who supposedly killed herself by jumping off a building at her prep school. The book is a mystery in the vein of *Gone Girl,* and both books feature a twist: At the end of *Reconstructing Amelia* it's revealed that Amelia didn't jump; she was pushed. In the book, nothing is as it seems.

This book's presence on the roof of the parking garage remains confusing to her family and friends. (Her parents haven't read the book, only the synopsis.) Did Madison want them to comb through her past to try to piece together the different versions of her, to come to some logical solution for why she had jumped off the building? And that final twist at the end of the book: Was that just an inconvenient detail that didn't fit into Madison's story, but since so much else about the book did fit—Amelia was even Madison's confirmation name—she was willing to overlook the ill-fitting ending? Or was she figuratively trying to say that Madison felt she, too, had been pushed?

Maybe all Madison was trying to say was that she saw a version of herself in Amelia, in the perfectly crafted veneer that could never feel like an honest reflection of her interior life. Just as Madison worried that she could never find validation for her struggle, because how could someone so beautiful, so seemingly put together, be unhappy? This is illogical, of course, like believing a computer's hard drive can't break simply because the screen hasn't a scratch.

Depression does not have a one-size-fits-all prognosis. Bill Schmitz Jr., the former president of the American Association of Suicidology, points out that the course varies. "In a way, it's the same as cancer," he says. "For some, we might prolong life for months, for years. For others, it can be very sudden."

Madison left the bag of gifts out in the open, where she knew it would be found, then walked away from it. The farther she got from the bag, the farther from any connection to her family, her friends, and to the life she had just started to live.

There are friends and family who believe Madison took a running leap over the metal railing, clearing the side as she had once cleared hurdles on the track. She landed in the bike lane some distance from the side of the building, which seems to suggest a momentum that could not have been gained from standing on the edge, looking down, and dropping. If she'd taken a running leap, then Maddy never had to stare at the ground, truly contemplate it, before choosing to let go.

Maybe she meant to jump. But then, maybe she didn't truly understand. Then again, maybe she did. "People do a lot of different research before doing this," Emma says. "And if you run and jump, it just happens. It's over with. And you don't have to struggle. I just can picture her walking up there and knowing that she could jump, just setting her mind to it and knowing it could happen—that's something I can see her doing. When she gets on that line in track, it's like: 'I'm doing this.' She was so determined with everything that she did, maybe even too determined. That's not the greatest way that people should be. But that was something about her."

"I've thought about what that must have felt like, being up there," says Jackie Reyneke. "That's something that's scary to me, looking down. When I'm at an amusement park, at the top of a Ferris wheel or roller coaster, and I look down, I always think, 'How could she have done that?'"

The first responders found the gifts with the following note:

> *I thought how unpleasant it is to be locked out, and I thought how it is worse perhaps to be locked in. For you mom . . . the necklaces . . . for you, Nana & Papa . . . Gingersnaps (always reminds me of you) . . . For you Ingrid . . . The Happiness Project. And Dad . . . the Godiva chocolate truffles. I love you all . . . I'm sorry. I love you.*

The first sentence of Madison's note is a quote from Virginia Woolf, who drowned herself at the age of fifty-nine.

The last thing Stacy Holleran texted her daughter was an update on how the family's youngest, Brendan, had performed at his track meet. At 7:35 p.m., she wrote: "B came in 2nd in 4x4." About two hours later, as Stacy was collecting Brendan from Highlands, a call came in to Stacy's cell phone from a 215 area code: Philadelphia. The call was from Steve Dolan. "My phone rings, and I answer by saying, 'Is Madison okay?'" recalls Stacy. "Something didn't feel right: Why is he calling me so late on a Friday night? And he just didn't know what to say—I think he assumed I had gotten a call already. I think he was calling to say he was sorry, and he paused. He thought the police or school had already called. So he's like, 'I heard something happened to Madison, but I'll find out more details and call you back.'"

Shaking, Stacy hung up and immediately called her husband. After that, she called Ingrid.

"Are you with Madison?" Stacy asked.

"No, I haven't heard from her," Ingrid said.

Stacy explained the call she had just received, then asked, "Who might she be with?"

Ingrid said she wasn't sure, that she hadn't heard from Madison in hours, and that Maddy was supposed to have met some people at the Penn cafeteria but hadn't shown. Ingrid said she would go over to Madison's dorm and call Emily, Maddy's roommate.

While Stacy was talking to Ingrid, Jim was talking to Ashley, who was back at school in Alabama.

"Have you talked to Madison?" he asked.

"Yeah, I just talked to her, like, this afternoon—everything was fine," Ashley said. She had been on a group text with Maddy and Mackenzie; they were assessing the cuteness of a boy Ashley was considering going on a date with. *Do you guys think he's cute?* Ashley had typed. Madison responded: *Eh, debatable.* But when Ashley prodded her sister for more, writing, *Hellloooooooo?,* she hadn't heard back. That was in midafternoon.

"Well, try calling her," Jim said. "Her phone is dead."

Ashley called. No answer. But that wasn't unusual for Maddy. By that time of night her phone was often out of power and she was at a party anyway, and there was no way to connect with her until she got back to her dorm. Ashley logged on to Facebook and went to her sister's page. It said she was last active just a few hours earlier.

A few minutes later, Ashley's phone rang again. This time it was her mom. Stacy had just received another call from a 215 number: this one from the chaplain at Penn.

After hanging up with Stacy, Ingrid ran across campus to Hill, Maddy's dorm. Emily was there watching a movie with friends, in the room across from the one she shared with Maddy. That afternoon she had been at track practice, wondering, along with the rest of the team, where Maddy was. Emily knew that her roommate had switched her training plan, but she still found Madison's absence that afternoon unsettling. One of their teammates had asked Emily if she knew where Maddy might be, or when they could expect to see her, but Emily didn't know, so she just shrugged and said as much.

Around ten o'clock that evening, during the middle of the movie, Emily's phone rang. It was Ingrid. Emily looked at the caller ID. She knew of Ingrid only through Maddy, but she answered because she figured Ingrid would have a specific reason for calling.

"Hi," Emily said.

"Are you in your room?" Ingrid asked. She sounded panicked.

"No, I'm across the hall," Emily said.

"With Madison?" Ingrid asked.

"No, I haven't seen her."

"I need you to come down to the lobby," Ingrid said. Her voice was so even in its tone, without inflection, without emphasis on any specific word, that Emily's heart rate spiked. She stood up from the bed and walked downstairs to the lobby. Ingrid was standing there, phone in her shaking hand.

"You have to call your coach," Ingrid said. "You have to call him."

"I don't understand—why?" Emily asked.

"Something has happened to Madison," Ingrid said. "You have to call him."

"What—what do you mean—what happened?" Emily looked at her phone.

"I don't know, but we can't find her," Ingrid said. She seemed to know more than she was saying. "You have to call your coach."

"What? What do you mean?" Emily's first thought was that Maddy had tried to kill herself, but she couldn't really complete that idea.

"Please call your coach," Ingrid said.

Emily found Steve Dolan's number in her contacts and hit

the call button, but she didn't know what she would say when he answered—*I'm calling about Madison? I'm calling because I think maybe something happened to Madison?*

"Can *you* talk to him?" Emily asked as the call started ringing. "Because I don't know what's happening."

Emily handed the phone to Ingrid. Dolan answered.

"I'm calling about Madison..." Ingrid began.

Emily could hear her coach talking on the other end. She could also see Ingrid's hand shaking, her breath becoming irregular. A few seconds later Ingrid began crying hysterically, unable to hold on to the phone any longer.

Down in Alabama, Ashley's phone began to ring again.

"Mom," Ashley said. Then she realized that both her parents were on the line.

"She's gone," Stacy said. "She's gone, she's gone, she's... gone."

"What?" Ashley said. "Gone?"

"She's dead. Madison is dead."

"Oh my God."

Ashley walked into her roommate's room and told her what her parents had just said. Ashley shook her head: "I don't even know what's going on right now."

"What do you want to do?" her roommate asked.

"Let's go for a ride."

As the two drove around Tuscaloosa, the texts started

pouring into Ashley's phone. Then her grandpa called, crying. He had exchanged e-mails with Madison just a few weeks before:

On Friday, December 13, 2013:

I WANT TO KNOW AND I want to know the truth—HOW is Madison Holleran doing and I don't mean your grades.

I mean how are Y O U doing?

Answer quickly as I am old with not a lot of time left. Papa.

Madison responded the same day:

Date: Fri, Dec 13, 2013 at 3:29 PM
Subject: Re: YOU!

Never been worse

(The two spoke on the phone after this exchange.)

"Are you okay?" Papa now asked his middle granddaughter, because she seemed distant, stunned. "Yeah, I'm fine," Ashley replied, then looked at her hands, which she couldn't keep steady. "I don't understand what's happening."

"Coach?" Emily said, standing in the lobby of Hill.

Dolan repeated what he had just told Ingrid: Madison had

killed herself. He told Emily not to tell anyone else yet, because he needed to coordinate a way to inform everybody, in the correct way, and not have the information burn through the campus like an awful game of telephone.

"Yes, Coach," Emily said. "Okay, Coach."

She ended the call. The information didn't make sense. Emily didn't shout, or cry, or yell. She just stood there. *Maddy killed herself? But I just saw her. And now she's dead. How... why... what?*

Ingrid was a mess, inconsolable. The resident advisors who were on duty came to the lobby, and suddenly the space was filled with people, all wanting to know what had happened. The housing staff helped Ingrid and Emily to the lounge, calling Ingrid's roommate as they walked, asking if she could come to Hill and help with Ingrid.

An e-mail was sent out by the housing department to everyone who lived in Hill, letting them know that one of the students who lived in their dorm, Madison Holleran, had died. People started congregating in the lounge. The school's counseling services, CAPS, sent over employees to help. Because there were parties and events taking place all over campus, people started calling Emily to find out what had happened: Was it true?

At 12:41 a.m. Steve Dolan sent this e-mail:

From: Steve Dolan
Date: Sat, Jan. 18, 2014 at 12:41 AM

Subject: Urgent Message from Penn Track and Field

Dear Track and Field Family,

This is the hardest email I have ever had to write. It is with a heavy heart that I share with you the following information about your teammate and friend Madison Holleran.

In grief and sorrow we share the news that Madison Holleran (C '17) died Friday evening in Center City, Philadelphia. She was 19 and lived in Hill.

We will be having an emergency team meeting at 8:15 at the Dunning Coaches Center for all those who are not traveling on the early bus to tomorrow's meet. Coach Martin and I will be by our phones throughout the night if you have any questions or need or want to talk. I am on my way into the office, and will be there throughout the night.

Our numbers are below.

Emily stayed in the lounge at Hill until the sun was peeking over the horizon. Someone had pulled a mattress into the room across the hall from the one she had shared with Maddy. Emily slept there for a few nights so she wouldn't have to face what was behind the closed door.

"I put my phone away early that night," recalls Emma, who had been in her room at Boston College. "I woke up to a hundred text messages and calls. I was the last person to know. I was sound asleep; it was terrible. I called my mom right away. I had read my messages and I said, 'Mom, did Maddy die?' She was already on her way to come get me. I was like, 'It doesn't make any sense. I don't think she got murdered.' I started to realize she had done this to herself, because in my heart, nothing bad happened to her—I knew it wasn't something bad. Something clicked in my head that maybe suicide is what happened."

The Rules of Suicide

I am nervous. I'm waiting in a café in New York City, just around the corner from Columbia University. The décor is funky bohemian: tattered couches, lopsided coffee tables, lamps with jewel shades, beer in small cafeteria cups.

I'm nervous because any minute, Dese'Rae Stage will walk into the shop. I texted her that I've arrived at our agreed-upon location and that I'm sitting near the kitchen. The three dots immediately appeared on my iPhone—she was composing a response. *"Be right there,"* she wrote. A small part of me had hoped she would cancel. Conversations with strangers require focus, steady energy, the burden of making sure the conversation is efficient, never stalls, never becomes awkward. It's like going to the gym for a workout: until the moment it begins, you kind of hold out hope it won't.

But I'm mostly glad Dese'Rae is about to walk through the door. As a suicide survivor, she possesses insight I do not. She is a photographer, occasional writer, and suicide awareness activist. Stage's main project is called *Live Through This,* a portrait and oral history series on survivors of suicide attempts. The goal of the series is to humanize survivors, to shatter the stereotype about who lives with suicidal thoughts, and to change the conversation around suicide.

This last sentence—*changing the conversation*—is why I've asked Stage to meet me for coffee. We first met on Twitter in an exchange about how the American media—newspapers, magazines, documentaries, movies, even music—talks about suicide. The American Foundation for Suicide Prevention created a set of guidelines for how to write about suicide in a respectful way. And yet these guidelines are often ignored or manipulated, because they often deny our curiosity—that is, answering the who, what, where, why, when of a story.

Instead of This: Big or sensationalistic headlines, or prominent placement (e.g., "Kurt Cobain Used Shotgun to Commit Suicide").

Do This: Inform the audience without sensationalizing the suicide and minimize prominence (e.g., "Kurt Cobain Dead at 27").

Instead of This: Including photos/videos of the location or method of death, grieving family, friends, memorials or funerals.

Do This: Use school/work or family photos; include hotline logo or local crisis phone numbers.

Instead of This: Describing recent suicides as an "epidemic," "skyrocketing," or other strong terms.

Do This: Carefully investigate the most recent CDC data and use non-sensational words like "rise" or "higher."

Instead of This: Describing a suicide as inexplicable or without warning.

Do This: Most, but not all, people who die by suicide exhibit warning signs. Include the "Warning Signs" and "What to Do" sidebar in your article if possible.

Instead of This: "John Doe left a suicide note saying . . ."

Do This: "A note from the deceased was found and is being reviewed by the medical examiner."

Instead of This: Investigating and reporting on suicide similar to reporting on crimes.

Do This: Report on suicide as a public health issue.

Instead of This: Quoting/interviewing police or first responders about the causes of suicide.

Do This: Seek advice from suicide prevention experts.

Instead of This: Referring to suicide as "successful" or "unsuccessful" or a "failed attempt."

Do This: Describe as "died by suicide" or "completed" or "killed him/herself."

Stage walks through the door. I'm right in her line of sight, so she nods and walks over. We hug, even though this is the first time we've met. After a few minutes of small talk—she has just come from San Francisco, after an interview for *Live Through This*—we jump into the complicated topic of writing about, and talking about, suicide. To be clear: She does not speak for the entire community. Her opinions should not be considered chapter and verse, but rather one valuable viewpoint within a world of varying beliefs.

Kate: What kind of job does the U.S. do when it comes to discussing suicide?

Dese'Rae: We're a country full of rubberneckers, you know? So when suicide comes up, we're either going to make a joke about it, have it be the punch line, or with writers, it's often hyperfocused on the precise moment of death: "This is what happened, here is who saw it, here's how it felt to see it, this is the way in which the blood splattered." And rarely does this kind of coverage get to the core of the issue: How was this person feeling? How can we change it? Why is this happening?

Kate: Throughout human history, storytelling has provided comfort. How do you balance that fact with the idea that, when it comes to suicide, too much storytelling can be gratuitous and dangerous in perpetuating myths about suicide?

Dese'Rae: They're not mutually exclusive: good storytelling and humane storytelling. What's not happening right now, that needs to happen more, is writers asking themselves what insight a certain detail actually offers the reader. For example, publishing a suicide note. What insight is that giving us into that person other than how they felt in, possibly, the toughest moment of their life? Will publishing that note offer us much insight into the total person, or just fulfill a curiosity?

Kate: Okay, so I get your point about rubbernecking, but still I wonder...

Dese'Rae: And, to be clear, that isn't a judgment. I'm a super rubbernecker, too—we all are...

Kate: So what do you see as the concern around people reading these details and, as you say, rubbernecking?

Dese'Rae: Suicide notes, well—they're romantic, in a way, and also they're abnormal. I believe the latest statistic is that 18 percent of people leave suicide notes. So publishing a suicide note perpetuates the myth that everyone leaves one.

Kate: Oh, wow, just 18 percent? That's lower than I would have thought.

Dese'Rae: Right! Most people don't leave suicide notes. So there is that. And suicide notes give us this feeling that we're going into those last moments and really feeling that moment and basking in its sadness and its tragedy. But, also, because of that, a suicide note anchors us in that single moment. It does not focus our attention on the more important areas: the beyond, in both directions, the before and after this single moment. What leads up to it and what comes after—does the suicide note offer us insight into any of that? No, we focus on the suicide. I don't think enough people realize that suicide is something that is cumulative, and there are certain catalysts. And in our storytelling, we often need to find one specific reason. It's much, much more complicated and you're never going to boil it down to a single headline.

Kate: Why are the guidelines the way they are?

Dese'Rae: Truth is, suicide prevention is a young field. I mean, Edwin Shneidman pioneered this field and opened the first suicide prevention center in 1958. That's not that long ago. So we're still trying to gather information so that we can make better decisions and recommendations. First, we need to find out exactly how suicide is talked about in popular culture and everyday life. I've started logging any reference to suicide I see in pop culture. Not through Google searches, which would require me to seek it out, but just organic references to suicide. I want to understand where we're coming from as a culture. People often say: "We don't talk about suicide." That's actually not true. We are talking about it. It's just that we're talking about it, often, in really unhelpful ways.

Kate: Can I have an example?

Dese'Rae: For example, in our TV shows, there are constant references to suicide, but they're almost always jokes. And that's not to say I don't have a sense of humor about suicide—doing this work you kind of have to—but on TV, the people making these jokes and writing these jokes don't seem to have thoughtfully considered suicide. They're just throwing something out there halfheartedly, in the hopes of getting a laugh. My concern is that if this is how we're thinking about and portraying suicide—as something someone might do just because they got broken up with—then how can we get people to care about it in a meaningful way, one that might change the suicide rate, or change the funding?

Kate: And how often are we speaking about suicide in a sophisticated way?

Dese'Rae: Not often. One example of when it was handled really well was the movie *Skeleton Twins*. It's funny and it's sad, and there's a part in it that's scary: a graphic depiction of a suicide attempt. But these characters feel relatable and three-dimensional. The thing for me about suicide is all about relatability: if we can relate to the people who have been through it, then maybe we're going to care. But if we're constantly jabbering in a distant way, as if these aren't real people—your friends, your neighbors, your family members—how are we going to get anywhere?

Kate: Sometimes, I think, a lot of people don't want to talk about suicide in a real, sophisticated way because it's just too scary.

Dese'Rae: Oh, absolutely, I get that. I think that's why some professionals didn't want to hear from people like me, from living survivors, for so long. Because then it was like, "Oh, now I'm being faced with this thing—literally in my face. This human is in front of me and they tried to kill themselves and what does that mean?" That is scary on so many levels. What I try to do in my work is show the depth and breadth of people who experience this—and it's scary, but denying its existence isn't helping anybody. So how can we talk about it in a safe way? I think letting people who have been through it talk openly and matter-of-factly is helpful. There is research that proves that exposure to people with mental health issues is hugely impactful on the attitudes of everyone around them. This might be common sense, but everyday people sharing their stories is even more important than celebrities using their platforms.

Kate: How do we satisfy the need to talk about suicide openly, but to not encourage clusters, or copy-cat suicides?

Dese'Rae: I would like to imagine that the silence, or the inability to talk about it in healthy ways, directly relates to more suicides. I'm concerned when I see a kid kill themselves, and in the aftermath, we say, "Oh, if we plant a tree, that romanticizes the fact they died, so let's not talk about it at all, 'cause why did they do that?" It doesn't have to be that way. People die by suicide, and they were people and we loved them, so honor them. There is a line between honoring and romanticizing what happened.

Kate: When it comes to suicide, why do we become so preoccupied with finding a "why"?

Dese'Rae: If it's cancer, it's scary, but we can deal with it and there is usually a game plan. If it's suicide, it could be any number of things, or a mixture of things, or years of traumas—all kinds of stuff. You can't pinpoint it, and I think that's what's scary. So looking for the "why?" is about answering the question "How do I avoid this thing happening to me? How can I avoid it?" But the truth is, you can't. If you do, it's simply because you're lucky.

Kate: How can we be more responsible when talking about suicide?

Dese'Rae: The question is: Is the act the climax? I don't think it is. Say, my story: I experienced an acutely bad two years and I made a decision one day based on a catalyst and I took some pills and I drank some stuff, and I tried to cut myself. Now, is that the interesting part?

Kate: No. Now, right now, I want to know the acutely bad things.

Dese'Rae: Right. It's an abusive relationship; it's trauma; it's years of depression. It's a breakup with someone who is manipulative, someone who I could not get away from and didn't really want to. So that's the interesting part to me, because I want to dig into why people make decisions. That's the interesting part—it's about reframing the suicide story to be about the person's life, not just about their death.

CHAPTER 11

Shattered 11

Jim and Stacy could not believe what they'd been told on the phone. Maddy was not, could not be, gone. "Part of me was simply convinced: I don't think this is real; I don't think this happened," Jim says.

No logic existed to explain how Maddy's buoyancy, her spirit—eighteen years in the making—could be extinguished in one moment. Think of all the life that had been breathed into her: the hugs, the laughter, the birthday parties with friends, the Saturday morning car rides to soccer practice, the juice boxes and peanut butter and jelly sandwiches with the crusts cut off, the tears, the stern words, the I love yous, the endless list of things done for every loved child. So much energy poured into one being: their daughter.

This love, in bodily form, could not be erased from the world so quickly, could it?

Early the next morning, while Ashley was flying home from Alabama, Jim sat in the car, stunned. His good friends drove him to the medical examiner's office in Philadelphia. The head of security for Penn was there, too. And so were two Philly police officers. There, he was shown a photo of his daughter's body, confirming that no mistake had been made, though really the photo felt like proof that a million mistakes had been made. He was also given the toxicology report. Madison had been sober, not a drop of alcohol in her blood—a fact that seems reassuring at first, but quickly becomes soul-crushing.

Maddy did not look dead. She looked like she was sleeping. And this felt like a small kindness, though such kindnesses often shatter a cracked heart.

At the examiner's office Jim received Maddy's offering, the bag of gifts she had left for her family. The small tokens of love and explanation summoned a dangerous cocktail of emotions. Jim found the picture of Maddy as a kid. He pulled it out of the book, held it. "She had shown me that picture over break, while she was home, and she goes, 'I want this picture,' and I was like, 'Why?' It's just this cute picture of her holding a tennis racquet when she's six years old, and she's like, 'I want to put it in my room in my collage.' So maybe it was little things like that that made me think she had been planning this. We had no idea, it was just seeing that picture, and it being there among everything, that made me wonder."

"I'm still confused about that bag of gifts," Jim said later. "I mean, the time and the effort that it appears she put into it, that maybe she planned this and to go ahead and, in her greatest time of need, still be thinking of others. It's just, it's unbelievable."

Jim needed to go to the parking garage. He had to see where his daughter had died. He had to know what the building looked like, what his daughter had seen in her final moments, how she could have decided to let go — so literally. "Seeing is believing," he says. "And I couldn't believe it, so I had to see everything."

He did not go alone. His friends went with him to the corner of 15th and Spruce. They walked to the top of the garage: nine flights. Jim stepped into the pain of knowing, of seeing through his daughter's eyes. He walked to the railing and looked down. He kept looking. He allowed himself to picture what Maddy had seen just hours before. He imagined the fall, but he did not stop there. He imagined the hardness, the crushing stop. He let his mind hold these images for as long as he could, until they imprinted into his memory.

Jim turned to his friends and said: "I could not have done this."

Ashley Holleran arrived home about the same time as her dad. Jim had with him the crucial items the authorities thought they would want: Maddy's phone and her computer from her dorm room, as well as everything she had left atop the parking garage.

The house was already filling with people as the news spread through the community, and as Maddy's high school and college friends began making the pilgrimage to Allendale so they could all be near one another, so they could all try to make sense of the hole that had just been blasted into their hearts.

Nobody understood, Ashley especially, how one of their favorite people in the world had decided, so swiftly and suddenly, to leave them. Ashley had talked to Maddy every day, over text or on Facebook. She told herself that if anybody could have known, she should have. "I talked to her seven hours before she jumped," she said. "How did that not come up in conversation?"

Ashley wanted to look at Madison's computer. She was so thirsty for answers that she didn't allow herself time to feel anxious about what she might find. She felt she was working against a clock; that something could still be done to rewind what had happened. She had to find the thing that had set all this in motion so she could fix it, so she could say or do exactly what Maddy needed.

Ashley opened every message, most e-mails, and searched through the documents. But there was nothing. The only insight came from the absence of clues. Maddy had deleted

294 • WHAT MADE MADDY RUN

her Internet history. Whatever she had searched over the previous few weeks, she did not want seen by others. Or maybe it's possible that she routinely cleared her Internet cache, though that also seems unlikely. More likely, Ashley believed, was that Maddy had been researching methods for suicide and didn't want her family to know exactly what she had contemplated. Maybe, even at the end, she wanted to control her story. She was sharing some thoughts—in the notes, in the choice of gifts—about why she had made this choice. Her family didn't need to know the desperate thinking that had gone into what looked like a tidy ending. This thinking was, in a striking way, similar to the concept of the Penn Face, the idea that most students at Penn aimed to project a calm, collected, placid exterior, while beneath the surface they were furiously pedaling to stay afloat. Even in her suicide, which seemed to convey the message that life had overwhelmed her, Maddy apparently still cared about projecting a collected, determined image.

Ashley had launched Maddy's iMessages, and since the computer had automatically connected to the house's wireless, and since Maddy's cell number was still active, the application began processing the text messages that were still coming in. At first the hundreds of texts were asking if she was okay, asking her to please text back, to call, that a horrible rumor was going around.

Then came a different kind of text: searching, heartbroken.

— I love you. God rest your soul.

— I'll miss you Madison. More than you knew.

— I just don't get it mad. You had it all.

— I'm sorry if you needed more from me. I had no idea.

— But I loved you like no one else. Just know that.

Part of the grieving process, that's what these were—the opening days. And this behavior was no different from that exhibited by the brokenhearted over the years. They continued to communicate with Madison the way they always had. Maddy had always been in their phones when she wasn't there in person, and so for a fleeting moment they could convince themselves that nothing at all had changed. She was just somewhere else, as usual, and they could just write her a text.

Everyone seemed to have a piece, an insight, an anecdote, that illuminated some aspect of their friend that others had never seen. The kids from Penn drove to New Jersey, where they met the kids from Allendale, her lifelong friends. "It was a pretty crazy experience," says Ashley Montgomery. "It was almost like we were putting together a puzzle of somebody's full life, like all the pieces were kind of coming together, and I think that was maybe more for me than her high school friends that it felt that way. I had only been with her through the college chapter of our lives, a few months of it, anyway.

To actually hear people say, 'Yeah, this is how she was here,' was just really interesting. But the fact was, I knew she was a great person when I met her, but I didn't see as distinct of a change because there hadn't been the experience with 'the old her'—the 'her' at home."

Oddly, the transition to college was both the trigger for depression and the reason she could hide her pain so well. Picture Madison walking a bridge connecting Allendale to Philadelphia. She looks down and notices how high she is; she looks across and notices how far there still is to go; she looks back, longingly, but that direction is no longer accessible to her. She takes a deep breath. She stops, rests on her knees, sweat dripping from her brow. This journey is longer and harder than she thought. And when she arrives in Philly, the walk has stripped her of a layer of buoyancy. Yet nobody in Philly notices the change, because they have never before met Maddy—any version at all. And you can only spot the after if you've known the before.

Some crossover between Maddy's worlds existed, but not much. And those who had known her when she was a kid, and noticed a shift in behavior once she got to college, could not see the change happening. As her friends sat together swapping stories, they realized that no one person knew enough to have helped Maddy. Perhaps a boyfriend, a partner, might have been the person intimate enough to see all the warning signs. In fact, it was one of Maddy's ex-boyfriends from high school who may have possessed a clue that even Ashley

Holleran hadn't known: "He told me, 'Madison started going to church at Penn.' And I was like, 'What?' I said, 'She never did that in high school.' My dad goes to church all the time, and if anyone would go with him, it was usually me, but not really anyone else in my family. So when he said, 'Yeah, she started going during the fall semester,' I thought to myself: *She never told me that, or anyone else, really, except for him.* He said, 'I don't know, she just said that she felt comforted by it; that it helped her.' And I guess, in retrospect, that does make sense."

More than two years after Madison's death, Ashley still can't quite wrap her mind around the dearth of answers. "I kept thinking there was definitely more to this," she says. "I just felt like there was a secret or something, like someone must have known, that one specific thing had happened, that she had told someone about her plan. I just kept wishing I knew the extent of everything, but obviously I can't ask her. So now I know that I'm not going to know. And I guess I've just kind of accepted that."

About a year after Madison's death, one of her teammates decided to quit the track team. She sent the following explanation to her teammates and included Maddy's e-mail address among those who received the message:

> I don't want to bore all of you with the nitty gritty details of
> why I ultimately decided to leave, but I thought I owed it to my

teammates to give some sort of explanation...Like some of you know, for a large part of my freshman year I was really, really sick and was on and off running for a while because of that...I went into summer with a new and excited mentality about running, and I faced new health problems so my training was pretty spotty. Obviously for a while I felt really discouraged about my running, and going to practice became something I stressed out about rather than something I looked forward to. And unfortunately, as I have finally started to come back every day to practice to run, I feel the same way more than ever. And if there is any positive message I have taken away from the tragic weekend with Madison, it's that we need to do what makes us happy.

I've realized that there are a lot of things I want to take advantage of during my time here at Penn, and I want running to continue to be something I love, not something that stresses me out or ruins my health again.

Maybe "why" is not the question to ask about Madison's death. Or whether she deliberately chose this at all; that is, other than in the very moment she started climbing the stairs. A definitive story is needed for those of us left behind, so we can feel better. Amid chaos, order and understanding feel paramount. We feel we must find a reason for why she jumped— a reason that makes sense to a healthy mind.

But there is no one thing. There are rivers that merge and create a powerful current. And we can't fully know why they all merged, right then, right there, around Maddy. Still, we can try to analyze each one, the way it bends and curves, what it turns into when it blends with another. We can do this, learn everything we can, how to talk to others about their pain or our own, in the hope that fewer people get caught in this same, fierce swirl.

Acknowledgments

This book exists only because the Holleran family has placed the duty of public service above their pain. A thank-you to each of them, as well as to Madison's friends, who provided invaluable insight even while processing an unthinkable loss. To everyone I spoke with: thank you for your time and willingness to share. A special thank-you to Bob and Meg Weckworth, who knew and loved Maddy, and who now run the Madison Holleran Foundation: if not for them, the meaning behind this book would be muddled. Thanks also to Bob Gebbia and Christine Moutier of the American Foundation for Suicide Prevention for their guidance on how to respectfully tell Madison's story.

My own family and friends provided support throughout this process, offering advice and counsel when needed. My mom, Kathy, my dad, Chris, and my sister, Ryan, were generous with their time and energy, and the love of my life, Kathryn, heard me discuss the ideas in this book for two years and never fatigued. (I love you, GC.) Thanks to the team at Little, Brown, especially my editor, Vanessa Mobley, as well as Kait Boudah, Carina Guiterman, Ben Allen, Katharine Myers, and Craig Young, for believing in this book's importance, and to my agent, Michael Klein, who helped shepherd this story to the proper home. Many people helped shape this book, including Jay and Gay Lovinger, as well as my mom, who read everything I sent her within minutes. I am eternally grateful to my best friend, Shawna Hawes, for... everything, always. Last but not least, a huge thanks to espnW, specifically Alison Overholt and Laura Gentile, for shaping the original story, and for supporting me throughout this process.

Resources

Courtesy of To Write Love on Her Arms

Emergency Resources: Call 911

Crisis Text Line offers free 24/7 support for people in crisis. Within the United States, simply send a text to 741741. A trained crisis counselor receives the text and responds quickly. www.crisistextline.org

National Suicide Prevention Lifeline provides free and confidential emotional support to people in suicidal crisis or emotional distress twenty-four hours a day, seven days a week. 1-800-273-TALK (273-8255)
www.suicidepreventionlifeline.org

To Write Love on Her Arms (TWLOHA) is a nonprofit movement dedicated to presenting hope and finding help for people struggling with depression, addiction, self-injury, and suicide. TWLOHA exists to encourage, inform, and inspire, and also to invest directly into treatment and recovery. www.twloha.com

About the Author

KATE FAGAN is a columnist and feature writer for espnW, ESPN.com, and *ESPN The Magazine.* She is a regular panelist on ESPN's *Around the Horn* and can also be seen on *Outside the Lines* and *SportsCenter.* Fagan spent three seasons covering the 76ers for the *Philadelphia Inquirer.* She is the author of a memoir, *The Reappearing Act,* and is cohost of the espnW podcast *Free Cookies.* Fagan lives in Brooklyn with her girlfriend, Kathryn Budig, and their two dogs.